Age-Proofing Your Brain, 2nd Edition

21 key factors *you* can control— to help you stay younger longer

Age-Proofing Your Brain, 2nd Edition

21 key factors *you* can control—to help you stay younger longer

Arlene R. Taylor PhD
Sharlet M. Briggs PhD

Success Resources International
Napa, California, USA

Age-Proofing Your Brain, 2nd Edition

Address requests for information to:

www.ArleneTaylor.org
www.SharletBriggs.com
www.LongevityLifestyleMatters.com

ISBN # 1-887307-85-0

Special thanks to: Michelle Nash, David H. Hegarty, Brenda L. Balding, and Margie Penkala

Illustrations: www.openclipart.org; Arlene R. Taylor; Seth Foley at sfoleystudios@aol.com

Cover design and production: David O. Eastman

Printed in the USA

Dedication

Age-Proofing Your Brain is dedicated to people all over the world who have asked questions such as:

- Are there any factors within my control that can help my brain stay young longer?

- Are there any studies that can provide a roadmap for a more successful and graceful growing-older journey?

- Are there preventable things I clearly need to avoid?

- Are there steps I can take to preserve my brain function for as long as possible?

In this, the age of the brain, the answers are yes, yes, yes, and yes.

Researching the information and writing this book has undoubtedly helped to stimulate and preserve ours. Brains, that is. Thank you for asking!

Publisher's Reminder

You are responsible for your own choices, actions, thoughts, and behaviors. The authors have made all reasonable efforts to ensure that the information in this book is accurate and up-to-date. However, there are no representations or warranties provided regarding the information—expressed or implied.

The information and resources offered are for general educational and informational purposes only and do not present an in-depth treatment of specific research findings or topics. They are not intended to take the place of professional counseling, medical or psychological care, or recommendations from healthcare professionals.

Be sure to consult with your physician or healthcare professional before you make lifestyle changes or add physical exercising to your daily regimen.

The publisher, authors, and editors expressly disclaim all responsibility and any liability (direct or indirect) for adverse effects from the use or misuse of concepts presented herein.

If you find typos, please know they serve a purpose. Some brains really enjoy looking for mistakes—and making mistakes is part and parcel of being human.

Contents

The lifestyle you choose to live— including everything you eat, drink, think, say, and do or don't do—is a health-relevant behavior that self-medicates your brain either negatively or positively.

To achieve positive outcomes, make thoughtful lifestyle choices in the present with an eye to their impact on the future. Yours! To do that, keep learning.

Getting Started

The human brain is the most complex mass of protoplasm on earth—perhaps even in our galaxy.

Marian C. Diamond and Arnold B. Scheibel

 The coach watched as Leslie slouched into class—candy bar in one hand, soda in the other, hair uncombed, shoes untied, the very picture of 'don't care.' Glancing at the clock the coach was tempted to make a comment but refrained from doing so in front of the other students.

The opportunity to catch Leslie alone came at the second break. "The way you're going will adversely impact your brain and immune system, which will impact your success in this sport," said the coach.

"What does *adversely* mean?" asked Leslie, insolently.

"Harmful, negative, unhelpful, likely to cause problems," said the coach. "Two things working against each other."

"And *the way I'm going*?" Leslie was definitely confrontive.

"Your lifestyle," said the coach, "and how it is adversely impacting your success. Mindset, attitude, self-talk, sleep, exercise, nutrition, study, hard work, commitment—you know the drill. We've talked about it since the start of boot camp. As it stands now, if someone must be cut, talent notwithstanding, you'd be the first to go."

Leslie shrugged, took another large bite of candy and followed that with a swig of soda. "I'm doin' okay."

"What is your overall goal for this sport?" asked the coach.

"Olympic gold!" said Leslie promptly. "I want to be famous. I'm already better than a bunch of the others here so I can't see sweatin' the small stuff."

"Doin' okay won't get you Olympic gold," said the coach. "World class in any field is said to be 1 percent talent and 99 percent hard work. We're talking a minimum of 10,000 hours of wise, effective, practice. I believe you *do* have the raw talent but you obviously don't really want it very badly." Leslie's eyebrows shot up in a surprised face.

"Everything starts in the brain. Yours," said the coach. "That applies to success in this sport as well as to how long and how well you live while you're alive. Your mindset appears to be one of 'Get by. Do as little as possible. Trust your talent.' You may be a flash-in-the-pan. Olympic gold is a horse of a different color. I'm willing to coach you. But you, your brain and body, must do the work."

Leslie finished the candy bar and soda, then slowly turned and looked directly at the coach. "I don't know much about my brain or how to maintain long-term success."

"You and a lot of others," the coach replied. "Even in this the *Age of the Brain*, the mystery of the human brain is just that for most people—a mystery. Fortunately, research is demystifying at least some of that."

"How much do *you* know about the brain?" asked Leslie, somewhat argumentatively, one eyebrow raised.

"I'm learning," said the coach, smiling. "I do know the brain can only do what it thinks it can do. If you think you can or you think you can't, you're right. And your mindset impacts your body, immune system, health, success, and even your potential longevity."

Leslie stood looking at the ground for a long time and finally said, "I love this sport. Honestly I do. But I think I've been afraid I couldn't achieve what I really want, so I just pretended not to care. But I *do* care. I'd like your help to craft the mindset and lifestyle that will help me succeed."

"You have it," said the coach. "First, be on time. Second, lose the candy and soda. Third, attend every session I present, especially those on brain function. And last but not least, start thinking *can-do*." Leslie nodded and actually squeezed out what just possibly was a small smile.

Neuroscience

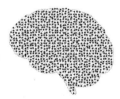

In 1995 Richard D. Broadwell, editor of the journal *Neuroscience,* wrote:

> *We sit on the threshold of important new advances in neuroscience that will yield increased understanding of how the brain functions and of more effective treatments to heal brain disorders and diseases. How the brain behaves in health and disease may well be the most important question in our lifetime.*

Broadwell nailed it. A great deal has been uncovered about brain function in the intervening years since 1995. And what has been learned can help *you* age-proof your brain.

Up until the last part of the 20th Century, much of what was known about the brain was discovered somewhat indirectly (e.g., observation of behaviors, studying the anatomy of a brain post-mortem, and evaluating tests from blood and cerebral-spinal fluid). In the 21st Century, 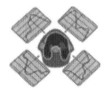 however, new state-of-the-art testing modalities for brain-function research are opening up the brain much as ocean-going ships once opened up the globe. Information related to brain function is now available in most countries in a plethora of formats. The types of brain scans continue to proliferate and what they reveal is indeed revolutionizing the knowledge about brain function.

Amazing, the human brain. It is estimated to have about a hundred billion neurons or nerve cells and maybe even more supporting glial cells, two million miles of axons, and a million billion synapses, making it the most complex structure, natural or artificial, on earth. In thirty seconds it likely produces as much data as the Hubble Space Telescope has produced in its lifetime.

How much do you know about your brain and how it functions?

No surprise if your answer is, "Well, I know I have one, but that's about it." To millions of people word-wide the human brain is a puzzle. Tim Green and colleagues put it well in an article that was published in the journal *Neuron*.

What seems astonishing is that a mere three-pound object, made of the same atoms that constitute everything else under the sun, is capable of directing virtually everything that humans have done: flying to the moon and hitting seventy home runs, writing Hamlet and building the Taj Mahal— even unlocking the secrets of the brain itself.

A vital body without a vital brain, however, is somewhat meaningless in terms of quality-of-life. Living longer in and of itself is not necessarily desirable unless your brain remains up to snuff. And you play a role in keeping it up to snuff. The way in which your brain functions impacts not only who you are innately but also everything you think, say, and do, including your level of health and your potential longevity.

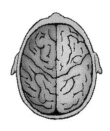 In this, the *Age of the Brain,* studies have shown that some age-related brain deficits can be prevented and some even reversed. This means that to a much larger extent than previously believed, you control how healthy you are, how long you are going to live, and how well your brain functions while you are alive. You are the only one who can age-proof your brain. Even if you cannot do everything, you *can* do something! And it's important. Brain function is associated with health and potential longevity.

As Tony Robbins put it:

To be or not to be isn't the question. The question is how to prolong being.

The Immune System

Enter the immune system. Your brain has a profound impact on your immune system and the way in which it functions. "The what?" you may ask. Your immune system. How much do you know about your immune system and how it functions?

For many, the human body's immune system is even more of a deep dark hole than the brain. As with the brain, immune system function is associated with health and potential longevity—just in a different way.

It is virtually impossible to separate the brain from the body and brain health from body health. Candice B. Pert PhD was recipient of the first-time award of the Theophrastus Paracelsus Foundation in Holistic Medicine, Switzerland. Recognized for her pioneering work in the area of Psychoneuroimmunology or PNI, Dr. Pert coined the term *BodyMind* to describe the close brain-body connection. This means that improved brain health tends to goes hand-in-hand or hand-in-glove with improved body health. That's one good reason for doing everything you can to support both your brain and immune system.

Think of the brain and the immune system as collaborators. The health of the brain and the health of the immune system are linked. Metaphorically, their hands are shoved so deeply in each other's pockets it's often hard to tell which is which—as one researcher put it. The old hand-in-glove metaphor works well, too. What is good for the brain is also good for the immune system. Take care of one and the other benefits, as well.

The brain-immune system connection is far more than metaphorical, however. In what has been termed a "stunning discovery that overturns decades of textbook teaching," researchers at the University of Virginia, School of Medicine, recently found that the brain is directly connected to the immune system by lymph vessels that run through the meninges (see drawing below), three protective membranes that cover the human brain. Previously these lymph vessels were not thought not to exist in the meninges. According to Jonathan Kipnis, a professor in the Department of Neuroscience and director of the Center for Brain Immunology and Glia, this discovery "changes entirely the way we perceive the neuro-immune interaction."

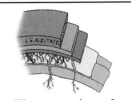

Three meningeal membranes between the skull on the top and brain tissue on the bottom

When you take responsibility for age-proofing your brain, you may be able to age-proof your immune system at the same time. You'll be glad you did. So will everyone who knows you! Staying healthy and growing older gracefully may be the best gift you can give to the next generation. Naturally starting early is ideal. Nevertheless it is rarely too late to create and live a high-level-healthiness lifestyle.

Most people have at least a general idea where their brain is housed (smile) even if they know little about how it really functions and what they can do to support and impact it positively. Far fewer can name the organs and tissues that comprise their immune system or where they are located throughout the body.

The drawing below shows some of the organs and tissues that generally are believed to comprise the immune system—some of which may surprise you. The immune system also includes miles (or kilometers) of lymph vessels that would circle the globe several times if laid end to end and that connect the hundreds of lymph nodes.

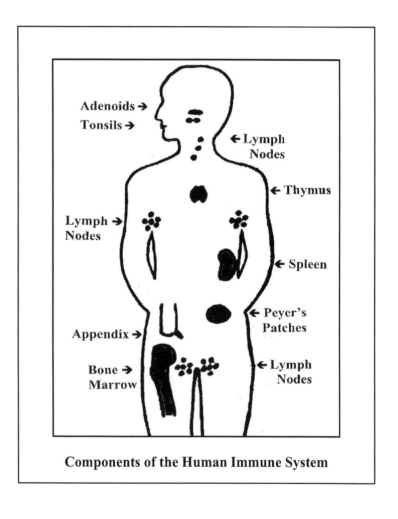

Components of the Human Immune System

Key Factors

Age-Proofing Your Brain addresses twenty-one key factors that have been found to impact the process of growing older and over which you have partial if not complete control—often more control than you might realize.

Brain-function information related to each key factor is included as well as 'Be Brain Wise' tips to help you age-proof your brain. The more factors you identify, learn about, and take responsibility for managing effectively, the more likely you are to develop a high-level-healthiness lifestyle—or a Longevity Lifestyle—and live it for as long as you live. The Selected Bibliography contains additional resources, should you desire to study more, as does the Authors & Resources section.

As William Arthur Ward put it:

If you can imagine it, you can achieve it. If you can dream it, you can become it.

Your brain is your greatest resource. Do everything in your power to keep it healthy, happy, motivated, and functional.

Use it by design to have a long, happy, and healthy life—and leave this planet a better place than you found it. There are no guarantees. Life is unpredictable. The more consistently you do this, however, and the more brain-function factors you address, the more likely you are to retain a well-functioning brain—for longer.

An old proverb says:

> *You are the only person who can be yourself—no one else has the qualifications for that job.*

You are the only one who can age-proof your brain, too. Even if you cannot do everything, you *can* do something.

The problem is, as Soren Kierkegaard so elegantly put it:

> *Although life can be only understood backwards, it must be lived forward.*

This book is all about helping you live forward. Are human beings *too soon old and too late smart?* Perhaps. On the other hand, some humans do seem to be gaining ground in terms of healthiness and longevity.

Create a map for your brain to follow and picture yourself being successful. Be your best self. You and your brain are in this together, so enjoy the journey together and have fun. You only know what you know and what you don't know can cramp your style. Big time.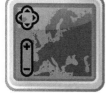

That's what this book is designed to do: share information that can help you increase your knowledge about your brain and your immune system and the factors that impact your health and potential longevity.

No surprise, the first key factor is ***Nascent Knowledge.*** Turn the page.

—Getting Started

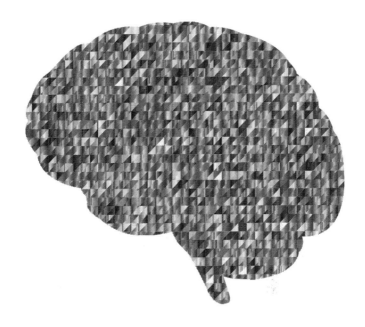

Be Brain Wise

It has been said that knowledge is power. Acquiring knowledge, especially that most elusive self-knowledge, requires awareness, intention, and a choice to learn. It is gained through learning from both education and your own life experiences.

In the words of Abigail Adams, however, 'learning is not attained by chance—it must be sought for with ardor and attended to with diligence.'

Key Factor—1
Nascent Knowledge

An investment in knowledge always pays the best interest.

—Benjamin Franklin (1706-1790)

 "The news this morning talked about the *Age of the Brain,*" said Bill. "Said brain information is nascent, coming into its own. You know, brain scans and all that new stuff." He kicked the tires on his friend's car. "Running out of tread, Jim," Bill said. "You and your tires." Jim laughed.

"I'm reading a book about brain function and learning some fascinating information," Bill continued "It's helping me better understand some of the choices I've made, explains how to communicate more clearly with myself and others, and offers tips for how to stay healthier and younger for longer. That alone is worth its weight in gold!"

Jim looked at Bill, "You're serious about this!" Jim said.

"I am serious," said Bill. "I'm also having fun. I figured I had some neurons, thinking cells, in my brain because I know two and two make four." He laughed. "But I had no idea neurons were also in my heart and gastrointestinal tract. I *think* with my heart and my gut, for heaven's sake. Who knew?"

"Guess you only know what you know," said Jim.

"I'm starting to realize that what I don't know is often the spoke in the wheel of my life," said Bill. "My gut is in turmoil half the time. I'm getting the picture that I could probably give it a break—my gut—by choosing to *think* differently."

Knowledge can be defined as facts, information, and skills acquired by a person through experience or education. Acquiring it is a process, developed by learning, by experience through practical application, and by evaluating the outcome and whether it was negative or positive. Humans have been interested in the brain for eons. New testing modalities are helping to shed light on what has been dubbed the most amazing chunk of biological real estate in the known universe. And what brain researchers are discovering is not only helpful but also exciting.

Your knowledge—what you know or don't know and how you apply it—profoundly impacts your brain's health: its ability to be alert, pay attention, think quickly and efficiently, combat fatigue, and store and reconstruct memories. The knowledge you possess has a great deal to do with the lifestyle you chose, which impacts your level of health and wellness, how efficiently and effectively your brain functions, and even your potential longevity. The good news? You can learn what is being discovered about the brain and the immune system.

Knowledge is one thing, of course. The practical application of what you know on a daily basis is another. Use brain-function information to expand your knowledge and to craft and implement practical applications that work for you.

Your Brain Is Unique

Human brains are more alike than they are different, regardless of race, gender, or culture. Brain tissue is the same color regardless of the skin tones on the body that houses the brain. And each brain develops uniquely. This means that no two brains on this planet are identical in structure, function, or perception—not even the brains of identical twins! Furthermore, each brain becomes more unique as it gets older because every thought you think changes the brain—and no two brains every think identical thoughts. So get to know and honor your brain. No need to continually compare it with others. Hone your own. There isn't another like it on the planet!

Neurons

The human brain and nervous system contain billions of neurons, thinking cells, plus even more supporting glial cells. Brain neurons likely form the basis for your Intelligence Quotient or IQ, just one of many different types of intelligence. Many factors impact IQ (e.g., number of dendrites on each neuron, the connections between neurons, personal experiences, and learning from them—or not). And IQ is not just a static number. Some have suggested that you can raise your IQ between five and thirty points (depending on where you start) through an effective type of challenging mental exercise and rehearsal. If you dislike the IQ you currently possess, raise it.

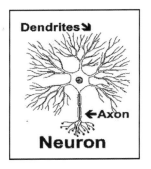

Your heart neurons, on the other hand, may form the basis for your Emotional Intelligence Quotient or EQ. High levels of EQ can help you use and apply your IQ much more effectively. As an aside, it appears that you may get your IQ potential from your opposite-gender parent. Avoid confusing that with whether or not your opposite-gender parent used their IQ to pursue formal education.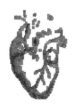

Researchers working with the ENIGMA project and lead by researcher Paul Thompson, a neurologist at the University of California, Los Angeles School of Medicine, reportedly have uncovered specific genes that are linked to both IQ and brain volume. Thompson has pointed out that brain size is not correlated with a person's intelligence. Einstein reportedly had a smaller than average brain but the number of connections between neurons was greater than average. (Decreased brain volume is sometimes seen in Alzheimer's disease, depression, obesity, and schizophrenia.)

Neurons in your brain and body generate electromagnetic energy or Em energy for short, a form of radiation energy (as are rays of the sun). Brain neurons may be arranged in fields of a million neurons per field, all vibrating at the same frequency within each field. Much like radio transmitters, they are able to send and receive their frequency potential. When you meet someone and perceive that you are on the same *wave length*, your brain may simply be recognizing frequency potentials. You have a sense of immediate connection. When not on the same *wave length*, you may not have a sense of connection, although you can still choose to be civil and kind, even though you may not want to spend much discretionary time with that particular brain.

Several bridges connect the two cerebral hemispheres. They consist of horizontal bundles of nerve axons, the corpus callosum being the largest. No hemispheric connections and your right hand wouldn't know what your left hand was doing and vice versa. Myelination involves the process of wrapping the nerve axons with insulation—think fiber optics. Myelination of the corpus callosum is thought to be completed about age twenty or twenty-one. Prior to that time the brain may be at risk for 'shorting out' and exhibiting behaviors that may lead more mature brains to exclaim, *"What were they thinking?"* Be patient, even calm, with brains that are 'not yet done.' Help younger brains understand the connection between choices and outcomes, decisions and consequences. Role model what you explain.

Multitasking and Miscellaneous

The brain can keep only one thought or task at a time in the foreground of consciousness, in what is commonly called working memory. Therefore, it is the rare brain that is able to do multitasking effectively. What appears to be multitasking is more likely just a series of rapidly alternating shifts of attention. Sanjay Gupta MD points out that likely you aren't actually doing multiple tasks at exactly the same time. You're just diverting your attention from one part of your brain to another part, which takes time and resources. Performance during multitasking is less efficient as compared to performing one task at a time. Some believe that a push toward multitasking may exacerbate ADHD (Attention Deficit Hyperactive Disorder) symptoms. Concentrating on only one task at a time is believed to be more effective and energy efficient.

Have you ever gone into another room to get something and then couldn't remember what it was you wanted? When you returned to the first room your brain reminded you of what you were looking for. Known as the Boundary Effect or Location-updating Effect, researchers believe this is because entering or exiting through a doorway serves as a type of event boundary for the brain, getting it ready to think about what is in the new room. Can you do anything about this? Sure. Let's say you want a stapler that's on your desk in another room. As you walk through the doorway into the second room, say aloud: "You are getting a stapler." That keeps what you want to get front and center in your brain's working memory and helps it to hang onto that thought as you pass through the doorway.

Fluid intelligence—that which demands speed when dealing with new or novel situations—tends to be better in young brains. Give yourself a little extra time when dealing with fluid intelligence in new or novel situations. Crystallized intelligence—specialized knowledge acquired from life experiences—is different. It requires large memory banks, recall, judgment, and good verbal abilities. Maturation can bring an advantage for crystallized intelligence. Hone it and affirm your brain for it.

Brain Stew Metaphor

In the culinary world, the taste of a stew is related to the type and amount of seasoning present. Think of your brain as a pot of chemical stew. Human beings continually self-medicate to alter their neurochemistry (to season their brain's chemical stew) and to make themselves feel better.

You can self-medicate by what you eat and drink, by ingesting medications and drugs (legal or illegal), and by everything you think and do. Make healthy decisions with an eye to the potential outcomes of your choices.

Expectations

The word expectation is commonly defined as a belief that something is going to happen or should happen in a specific way or is the most likely to happen. You've heard many of them, no doubt. Usually they erupt with some level of irritation, frustration, or disbelief, and once in a while with humor and laughter. It goes like this:

- "I do not understand her (or him)."
- "I cannot imagine what he (or she) was thinking!"
- "They should've been able to figure it out."
- "I have no idea what I was thinking."

Expectations can be deadly. Give up all expectations that another brain will understand yours. You don't even understand your own brain! The more knowledge you gain, however, the better you may understand brain function in general and something of yours in particular. Whatever you do, avoid meaningless argument and foolish controversy. All any brain has is its own opinion—which can change based on additional knowledge. Keep learning. Review what you learn. Some studies indicate that adult brains need to hear information three or four times to really move it into long-term memory.

The second key factor is ***Perspicacious Perspective.*** Turn to the next chapter and be prepared to honestly evaluate yours.

Be Brain Wise

Become mindfully aware of your own habitual choices and perspectives. For example, are you eating because you are physiologically hungry and your brain and body need food or are you eating because it's a habit or you are bored or because you are trying to feel better emotionally?

Make healthy choices and alter your behaviors as needed to help you achieve the consistently positive outcomes you desire and expect.

Identify and examine your perspectives about brain function and getting older. Unless you do this consciously you won't know whether your beliefs are appropriate, need tweaking, or warrant a major overhaul. If you have any negative perspectives, dump them, including Gerontophobia.

Multiple Ages

Human beings are a combination of several types of *ages*. Consider the following three types of ages.

> Your chronological age is unalterable. The fact is that you were born when you were born. You could lie about your birth date but lying is believed to suppress immune system function and you want to avoid that. Accept your chronological age as just a number and do what you can to live younger longer.

- Your psychological age can be changed. Most likely you know people who seem much younger, more mentally alert, and more vibrant than their chronological age. Of course, the reverse is also true.

- Your biological age can be speeded up or slowed down. Studies suggest you may be able to retard the onset of some symptoms associated with growing older. Embrace strategies to help you do this.

Ask yourself: how old would you be if you didn't know how old you were chronologically? Your perspective matters. Your mindset can impact your response to these ages.

Benign Senescence is a term for age-related forgetfulness, much of which is believed preventable. Tell yourself every day: "Janet, (or Joe) you are retaining your memory."

Read aloud for at least ten (10) minutes a day, hardcopy or electronic. Listen to audiobooks. Engage in stimulating brain activities for at least thirty (30) minutes a day. Play, have fun, and laugh. A lot! Build your vocabulary. While mental nimbleness for accessing words instantly can decline with age, your vocabulary can improve so you can grab a synonym.

Take a class at the local Junior College or by computer. Research in three countries has shown that for every year of education beyond basic college (or its equivalent) you reduce your risk of Alzheimer's by twenty (20) percent. Take advantage of on-line learning!

Assess your ability to interact with individuals of any age. Do you have a progressive and even entrepreneurial perspective, open to new information and its application? Are you able to think outside the box in relation to challenges in your world?

Believe in yourself. Do you give more weight to the opinions of others as compared to your own? According to Doctors Arnold Barry Fox in *Wake Up! You're Alive,* when you believe in yourself, brain circuits are open, allowing the knowledge and wisdom already there to circulate freely. Emotional channels open wide, allowing you to love and be loved, to enjoy life to the fullest. All your talents and skills are impacted by belief.

Life Satisfaction

Research by psychologist Bernice L. Neugarten related to adult development and growing older, identified the most important factor in a healthy process as your personal perspective of life satisfaction. The five most crucial ingredients for life satisfaction were identified as:

1. Enjoyment of daily activities
2. A positive mind-set (optimism)
3. A positive and worthwhile self-image
4. A belief that your life has meaning
5. Satisfactory achievement of major goals

Many individuals face challenges from societal myths and perspectives involving the worship of *youth*. Avoid getting sucked into them. Be especially wary of overemphasizing the advantages of youth. Prevent the desire for *youth* from interfering with successful living at every age and skewing your perception of the many benefits that can accompany meaningful maturation.

Quit believing that creativity is a relatively rare commodity rather than a mental faculty that every brain possesses. Activities that many judge as 'creative' are often rather narrowly defined according to—no surprise—personal perspective. Embrace creativity in your own way. Believe in it, hone it, honor it, enjoy it, and share it.

Stop adhering to a mandatory retirement age of sixty-five (reportedly set by German Chancellor Otto Von Bismarck) and allowing it to limit your life. It's *your* life, after all. What does an arbitrary number have to do with you?

Most people become aware of the need to care for their brain only when they begin to notice a decrease in brain function. You can prevent some problems, delay the development of others, and even reverse some. Get on board with prevention and be confident that you have done your best with the brain that has been leased to you for use on this planet. Develop a high-level-healthiness lifestyle to help delay the onset of symptoms of growing older. If you already have some symptoms, get busy with strategies to help reverse them. There is good news about this perspective.

- Those who take appropriate preventive steps may enjoy as many as ten additional quality years
  —Thomas T. Perls MD and Margery H. Silver EdD

- You can delay symptoms of aging by as much as thirty years by adopting a healthy lifestyle
  —Deepak Chopra MD

- Biologically we can reverse the aging process by fifteen to twenty-five years! —Miriam Nelson PhD

There's more good news. An article published in the journal Annals of Behavioral Medicine, August 2001, reported on studies of senior citizens who walked regularly compared to sedentary elderly. The studies showed improvement in memory skills, learning ability, concentration, and abstract reasoning. Stroke risk was reduced by fifty-seven percent in people who walked as little as twenty minutes a day.

Are you able to walk? What are you waiting for? Get moving! Sure, be realistic, but do what you can—every day!

Some individuals have the perspective that because they can no longer do what they used to do, it's all hopeless, a downhill slide to eventual oblivion. Others embrace a very different perspective; one that avoids allowing what you are unable to do to derail you from doing what you are able to do. They say things like:

- If you can't use a treadmill, try a reclining bike.
- If tennis is 'out,' try badminton or golf or walking.
- If you can't walk, swim.
- If you can't walk or swim, do chair exercises.
- If you're bedridden, breathe deeply ten times each hour and move whatever you can (e.g., rotate your ankles, pump your feet, and wave your arms).

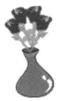

Abraham Lincoln's perspective was that you can complain because rose bushes have thorns or rejoice because thorn bushes have roses. Back to the glass half empty metaphor. George Carlin's perspective was that he sees a glass that's just twice as big as it needs to be.

In the main, one thing over which you have some control is your own perspective. Take a look at yours. If it is not helping you do what you *can* do purposefully, gracefully, and successfully, get busy and craft a perspective that does. Then for heaven's sake hang onto it and live it!

Key factor number three is ***Magic Mindset.*** To grasp the critical importance of mindset to age-proofing your brain, turn to the next chapter. It's waiting for you.

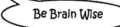

Be Brain Wise

Your mindset is a self-fulfilling prophecy that drives your self-talk and ultimately your behavioral choices. Set events in motion that can enhance your brain function, health, and happiness by developing and consistently implementing a positive can-do mindset.

Choose to think, believe, and speak in positive ways that lead to positive behaviors—which in turn promote health, happiness, and longevity.

Key Factor—3
Magic Mindset

The happiness of your life depends upon the quality of your thoughts.

—Marcus Antonius

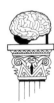 "I had a completely wretched appointment with my counselor today," said Pam, flopping into a recliner.

"What was so wretched about it?" asked her Aunt Jennie. "I thought you liked that counselor."

"I did—until today," said Pam. "Imagine telling a client that she needed a mindset readjustment. Imagine! For two cents I'd just quite school altogether."

"What did you say?" asked Aunt Jennie, trying not to smile.

"I told her that my grades had nothing to do with my mindset. If the teachers were any good I shouldn't have to study so hard. It's incompetent professors, that's what."

"I offered to have you live here so you could save money and have quiet undistracted time for study," Aunt Jennie said kindly. "It's mid-term, Pam, and you've hardly cracked a book, never mind skipping classes, partying until all hours of the night, losing sleep, and failing to turn in your assignments. Are you really going to blame your teachers?"

"Okay, so I've gotten off to a bit of a slow start," said Pam, smiling ruefully and having the grace to look at least a little embarrassed. "But I don't even know what a mindset is."

"Let's pull up a definition from the computer," said Aunt Jennie, booting up her laptop. "Here's one: a mental attitude, inclination, or disposition that predetermines a person's interpretations of situations and events and responses to them. Hmm-m." Pam shrugged and rolled her eyes.

"And here's something by Carol S. Dweck PhD, author of the book *Mindset.* According to her, there are *fixed* mindsets and growth mindsets. People with a fixed mindset believe that abilities are mostly innate and they tend to interpret failure as the lack of necessary basic abilities. They tend to believe that who they are is carved in stone. When they perceive failure, they feel worthless, unlucky, and often give up. On the other hand, people with a *growth* mindset believe that they can acquire any given ability and skill provided they invest effort or study. Even though they face challenges, growth-mindset people refrain from putting themselves down or throwing in the proverbial towel. They just keep on building their skills and practicing." Pam shrugged again but this time she did not roll her eyes.

"Dweck says that a growth mindset allows a person to live a less stressful and more successful life. Having a growth mindset doesn't force you to pursue something. It just tells you that you can develop your skills—it's still up to you whether you want to do that. I suppose it all boils down to whether or not you want to hit a bull's eye in life." This time Pam didn't even shrug.

"Oh, this is interesting," Aunt Jennie continued. *"Thinking* you are a failure or that you can't do something will contribute to you *feeling* like a failure. Your brain cannot do what it thinks it cannot do. If it does not perceive and expect success it will perceive and expect failure."

"But it's not as if I haven't been *trying*," said Pam, a definite whine in her voice.

"There's a huge difference between trying and doing," Aunt Jennie said, kindly. "Many *try*, while doubting success. *Trying* rarely achieves your goal. *Doing* often does because it means actually taking steps designed to increase your likelihood of success. Remember, your brain knows when you are serious and it gets on board to help you only when it senses you mean business. When it perceives you are in this only half-heartedly—in for a penny but not in for a pound— it fails metaphorically to put its shoulder to the wheel and just sits back waiting for you to resume your old habits."

"Using those definitions of trying versus doing, it's pretty clear I've been *trying* more than *doing,*" said Pam.

"So where do you want to go from here?" asked Aunt Jennie.

"I think I understand what my counselor was talking about," said Pam, straightening up in her chair. "I want a growth mindset and I'm working on it as we speak. We'll both be proud of my *doing* from here on out."

Your habitual mindset forms neural circuits in the brain that impact your attitudes, beliefs, and choices.

Choose Wisely

Is your current mindset helping you achieve your goals? Is it typically negative or positive, sad or happy, glad or mad, hopeless or hopeful? Your mindset has a great deal to do with the way in which you approach the aging process. The good news is that it is possible to change your mindset. Since your mindset style is learned, you can choose to develop a consistently positive mindset that can be much more effective—and if you choose to maintain that positive mindset, the brain can rewire itself to facilitate that attitude.

What type of mindsets did you observe during childhood? The conscious mind may be sabotaged by the more powerful subconscious mind as a direct result of early negative childhood programming and self-destructive behaviors. The more 'you can't' messages you received as a child, the more 'you can't' thoughts and experiences you may be having in adulthood.

Negativity Fallout

Negative thinking patterns can put your brain at risk for anxiety and depression and the resulting fallout. According to Doctors Arnold and Barry Fox, a negative thought is as dangerous as a physical germ. It can harm health, disrupt personal relationships, and contribute to failure. Negativity has been linked with neurotransmitter changes that can adversely impact both your brain and your body.

- Noradrenalin helps regulate mood. A sense of hopelessness is linked with lower levels of noradrenalin.

- Dopamine is essential for proper motor coordination and an ability to experience pleasure. Perceptions of being unable to cope are associated with decreased dopamine.

- Serotonin helps shape mood, energy levels, memory, outlook on life, and the experience of joy and contentment. Unmanaged anger, fear, and sadness are associated with lowered levels of serotonin.

Congruence and Energy

The brain wants congruence, wants everything to be in harmony and match. If your mindset is positive, your brain searches your memory banks for all the positive memories it can find and you can become even more positive. If, on the other hand, your mindset is negative, your brain searches for all the negative memories it can find and you will tend to become more and more negative.

A negative mindset can drain your energy, decrease self-esteem levels, increase anxiety and depression, suppress immune system function, and trigger the release of stress hormones that can adversely impact your brain and body over time. Jon Gordon wrote about it in his book *Become an Energy Addict:* "Think positively about the day ahead and you increase your mental and physical energy. Instead of being fearful and anxious, causing a release of stress hormones, thinking positively about the day will send positive energy to your body supplying you with sustained energy."

On the other hand, a positive mindset can promote optimum self-esteem, strengthen immune system function, contribute to high-level-wellness, and increase your available energy. A positive mindset asserts that for every problem there is a solution. When undesirable events occur, uncover the lesson to be learned, and look for the silver lining (typically there is one). The more you identify positive aspects and dwell on an increased understanding, the better your overall health will be. And that will further impact your choices and behaviors, especially related to longevity.

Health Relevance

Every thought you think is a health-relevant event. Meaning that your thoughts can move you toward or away from high-level-healthiness living; toward or away from health; toward or away from happiness and life satisfaction; toward or away from potential longevity. Studies have shown that the human brain prefers seeing happy faces. Picture yourself being happy. Negativity can be counteracted by using visualizations—mental imaging strategies that can actually rewire the way in which the brain works. Think positive thoughts; put a positive spin on every event to the extent possible. This sends messages to your brain that can be used to counteract negativity. It is not *Pollyanna*. It *is* choosing positivity!

Thoughts are just thoughts—and you have the power to change them if you choose to do so. Most people were never taught to correct the negative thoughts that swirl through their brains. Many things may trigger thoughts of fear, anger, or sadness. Pay attention and take appropriate action.

If you never question or challenge the negative thoughts that go through your brain, however, you may begin to believe them and hang onto them. Become aware of your thoughts. According to Oliver Wendell Holmes, Awareness is the first step on the continuum of positive change. When you become aware of sad, mad, anxious, or nervous thoughts, choose to think of something specific and positive. Tell your brain, "You are thinking about _____ (something positive)." You do not have to believe every thought that flits across your mind and you certainly do not have to hang onto and ponder it. This is important because thoughts lead to behaviors.

The title of a book by Peter McWilliams makes the point succinctly: *You Can't Afford the Luxury of a Negative Thought.* Take charge of your thoughts. If you have an *enemy outpost* of negativity inside your mind, get rid of it! It requires tremendous amounts of energy to staff an outpost. Use your energy to develop a positive mindset. Is a positive mindset magic? It's not *magic* and yet in a way it *is* magic, because it tells your brain what it can do—and your brain can only do what it thinks it can do. Patricia Neal put it this way:

> *A strong positive mental attitude will create more miracles than any wonder drug.*

The fourth key factor is something that contributes to one's success, although not everyone does it. Check out the next chapter, ***Affirmation Advantage,*** and learn how to gain an upper hand.

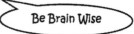

Be Brain Wise

The brain responds better to a specific communication style. The subconscious is highly receptive to simple, positive statements, so use that information to your advantage.

You are the only one who can program your brain positively for success. What are you waiting for? Time is passing. Consistently choose to think and speak affirmingly to help you be successful in living a high-level-healthiness lifestyle and age-proof your brain.

Key Factor—4
Affirmation Advantage

Mental states are particularly susceptible to affirmation.
Affirmation is the mind's programming language.

—Jean Marie Stine

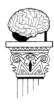 "I don't think I can do this, Doc," said Tallic, sighing. "I guess I thought it would be easier. I've told myself a hundred times, 'I don't want to drink sodas anymore because they're not good for my brain and my body.' And what do you think I do? I drink sodas."

"That is discouraging," said his doctor. "Telling yourself what you do *not* want to do, however, is unhelpful. Affirmations may be the most effective way to program your brain for success. They create a picture of what you want to accomplish in a specific situation or in an overall goal."

"Affirmations?" asked Tallic, frowning.

"Yes. Affirmations. A style of thinking and speaking that makes clear what you want to have happen instead of what you don't want to have happen. Tell yourself, 'Tallic, you are drinking water as your beverage of choice and you like the taste. You feel better. Avoiding sugar and artificial sweeteners is helping to age-proof my brain."

"Oh, I can do that," said Tallic. "Thanks, Doc."

Affirmation is a label for a powerful style of thinking that emphasizes using positive words to communicate with yourself and others. One of the three researched strategies that have been shown to enhance communication between the brain and the body, the other two are visualization (active mental picturing) and meditation (prayer being one form).

The brain creates internal pictures from thoughts and words and then follows them as a map. Think of affirmation as a tool to help you picture health and success and achieve it. Those internal pictures are perceived by your subconscious portions of the brain, which help move you toward your goal even when you are thinking consciously about something else. The affirmation formula is simple. Use short, positive, present-tense words and phrases. Speak as if you are already realizing your goal.

If you say, 'I'm going to ride my bike,' your brain recognizes the future tense. It thinks, *'When you get there I'll help you. Right now, I'm busy dealing with the present,'* and your goal stays just out of reach. When you speak as if what you want to do is already happening (e.g., Nell, you are riding your bike for thirty minutes), your brain recognizes the present tense and gets in gear to help you. It thinks, *'Okay, let's go. I'll help you.'* Thinking and talking about being a failure, will contribute to you *feeling* like a failure. Your brain can only do what it thinks it can do. If it does not perceive and expect success it will perceive and expect failure. Because your brain is very susceptible to an affirming style of communication, you can get ahead of the curve, in a sense, by learning to think and speak in positives. Talk only about what you are choosing to do.

Three Brain Layers

The brain can be described as three functional layers, each possessing distinct mental faculties that also continually interact with each other.

- The first or reptilian layer houses subconscious thought, including survival and instinctual-protective reflexes. It processes the present tense only. While it does not use language, it can perceive the internal mental pictures that language creates.

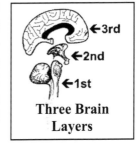

Three Brain Layers

- The second or mammalian layer also houses subconscious thought and contains the pain/pleasure center, directs immune system function, and can process past as well as present tenses. As with the first layer, although it doesn't use language it can perceive the internal mental pictures that words and thoughts create.

- The third layer or neocortex houses conscious rational and logical thought, uses language, and can process all tenses (present, past, and future). It can perceive both positive and negative statements, but it can have difficulty with negative thoughts and instructions because negatives represent a two-step process.

All brain layers can perceive positives quite easily because they tell the brain what to *do*—a one-step process. Your thoughts and words create the mental picture, your brain sees the picture, and understands what you want it to do.

Negatives represent the reverse of an idea, a two-step process that requires changing the first picture into a different picture. Negative statements tell your brain what not to do but not what to do. 'Don't think about the white bear' does not tell your brain what to think about. Is it supposed to think about a brown bear or a black bear or something else altogether?

When your brain hears the words '*don't touch the stove*,' it first pictures your hand touching the stove. It may miss the word *don't* or fail to recognize that this instruction actually means it is supposed to create and follow an opposite picture. On the other hand, when your brain hears '*keep your hands away from the stove,*' typically it first creates a picture of your hands apart from the stove. It is clear about what it is supposed to do. It can be difficult for the adult brain to imagine the reverse of an idea and a real challenge for a child's brain, especially if it involves abstract thinking.

Growing up did you hear more positives or negatives? If negatives, your brain is likely filled with negative pictures and messages. Using negatives may increase the likelihood that unhelpful pictures will circulate in the brain and your subconscious may try to help you achieve exactly the opposite of what you really want. Because all brain layers can perceive positives, using affirmations increases the likelihood that the desired pictures of what you want to have happen will filter down to the subconscious layers. Stop thinking and talking about what you do not want to have happen. Always think and speak in positives—a one-step process for the brain—to tell it exactly what you do want to have happen.

Price of Pejoratives

Avoid pejoratives even in jest. The third brain layer is able to understand a joke; the first and second layers probably cannot. When you say, "I feel a bad day coming on," your conscious mind may chuckle. Your subconscious mind may take that statement literally and oblige you by doing everything in its power to help you achieve 'a bad day,' whatever that means in your life. You cannot prevent all sad or bad events. You can have a leg-up on dealing with them. Affirmation is a tool that can help you deal appropriately with whatever happens.

Studies have shown that using your 'given name' and the word 'you' flips a switch in the cerebral cortex (thought center) and in the amygdala (seat of fear) that gives you psychological distance, enables self-control, and allows you to think clearly and to perform more competently. This style of speaking depersonalizes things a little and indicates that you and your brain—although separate entities—are working together. What you tell yourself and the words you use can make all the difference to your success. Use positive phrases with yourself and others, consistently:

- 'You remember' versus 'Don't Forget'
- 'You can' versus 'You can't'
- 'You choose' versus 'The devil made me do it'
- 'You speak softly' versus 'Don't yell'
- 'You are' versus 'I'm going to'

The brain wants congruence. It wants everything to match and be in harmony. When in the grip of a specific emotion, it tends to search for past memories with similar emotions.

Negative thoughts tend to trigger recall of negative memories, stressful thoughts of stressful memories, fearful thoughts of fearful memories, angry thoughts of angry memories, and so on. Of course positive thoughts tend to trigger recall of positive memories, which can help make life easier and even more enjoyable.

Some studies suggest that it is more effective to write out your affirmations and read them aloud several times a day. Reading aloud, as compared with repeating rote memorization, requires a different process in the brain and is believed to be much more stimulating. For example:

- (Name), you are enjoying brain exercises. They are an age-proofing strategy.

- (Name), you look and feel much younger than your chronological age. Life is good!

Willpower

Willpower is a function of the prefrontal cortex, that part of the brain directly behind your forehead. Although that portion of the brain is likely 'done' about mid to late twenties, hopefully you have been practicing using willpower correctly from very early childhood. Confucius said: "It is not that I do not know what to do; it is that I do not do what I know." Every human being struggles with that at some time or other in life. Once you have your affirmations in place and you are using positive self-talk, access willpower to follow-though on what you want to do.

According to Daniel M. Wegner PhD in his book *White Bears and Other Unwanted Thoughts,* willpower rarely works well to deprive yourself of something you already do for gratification, like trying to end a bad habit. Willing yourself *not* to do something just puts the thing you would like to avoid in working memory—the brain constantly thinks about it, which usually increases the behavior.

Willpower does work well to give you energy and perseverance to attain a goal, whether that be to develop a new behavior altogether or replace an old behavior with a healthier one. Stop talking about the old behavior or what you no longer want to do, and tell your brain what you are doing as if the new behavior is already in place—using affirmations.

Rather than saying, "I don't want to drink sodas anymore," try instead: 'Jeff, you are drinking water as your beverage of choice. You like the taste. You feel better.' Then access willpower to actually drink water as your beverage of choice.

Think of yourself as developing *skillpower.* That helps you make healthier choices. Then access *willpower* to help you follow through on those healthier choices. Use affirmations to tell your brain a positive story that will create a map for your brain to follow. In that way you begin to program your brain and immune system for health, wellness, and longevity. You are age-proofing your brain. You can do it!

The fifth key factor is **Active Mental picturing** or visualizing—although that word scares some. Turn the page and learn how to do this in a positive and empowering style.

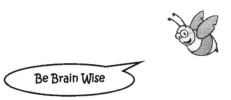

Be Brain Wise

Hone your brain's ability to recall and construct visual images within your mind's eye— internal mental pictures of what you want to achieve. Use virtual rehearsal to reinforce actual rehearsal or to prepare in advance when actual rehearsal is impossible.

Regularly picture yourself living a long time, with life in your years, and with high levels of mental, physical, emotional, and spiritual health. Others are doing it. You can too!

Key Factor—5
Active Mental Picturing

Visualize this thing you want. See it, feel it, believe in it.
Make your mental blueprint and begin.

—Robert Collier

"Okay, Sally,' said her father, helping her learn to ride a two-wheel bike. "This time I'll let go of the seat halfway from here to the open gate."

Everything went swimmingly until a neighbor's head rose above the fence, took in the situation, and called out: *"Don't run into the gate post, Sally."*

No surprise, Sally crashed into one of the gate posts. Her father hurried over to check that she was uninjured. "The neighbor told me not to hit the gate post and I ran right into it," said Sally, sniffling. "Maybe I can't ride a two-wheel bike after all." She sat dejectedly on the grass.

"Remember when we talked about the *white bear phenomenon?*" asked her father.

Sally nodded and said, "When you say, 'Don't think about the white bear,' I see a white bear in my mind's eye."

"Exactly," said her father. "Behaviors follow thoughts. And thoughts are just mental pictures in your brain."

"In fact," he continued, "Ralph Waldo Emerson said that you can't have an action without first having a thought—even if you're unaware of the thought. Saying 'Don't think about 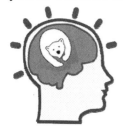 the white bear' actually puts a representation of a white bear into your brain's working memory. You picture it in your mind's eye and you will likely think about it even more frequently. A negative instruction tells you what not to do but doesn't tell you what to think about. When you heard the neighbor's talking head say, 'Don't run into the gate post,' what did you see in your mind's eye?"

Sally thought for a moment. "I saw myself running into the gate post with my bike." She laughed. "Crazy, crazy, crazy. I did just what I had been thinking about."

"Not crazy," said her father. "Commonly occurring. Now, listen carefully. 'Sally, ride your new bike right through the middle of the space between the two gate posts. Close your eyes. Can you see what you want your brain to do?" Sally nodded. "Now tell your brain: 'Sally, you are riding right through the middle of that space.'" Sally repeated it several times. "Okay," said her father. "Now, turn that picture into reality. Grab your bike. Let's go again. I'll help you get started. Be sure to tell your brain what you want it to do." This time, Sally rode her bike successfully right through the middle of the space between the two gate posts.

The human brain thinks in pictures. A thought is really just an internal mental picture. Visualizing is another name for the process of forming pictures in your mind's eye.

Your thoughts and words create a picture for your brain to follow—a map, as it were. Visualization can work as an extremely effective mind exercise. It is so powerful, in fact, that visualization is one of the three researched strategies that have been shown to enhance communication between the brain and the body (the other two strategies being affirmation and meditation).

In his book *Social Intelligence*, author Dr. Daniel Goleman explains visualization as mental rehearsal:

> *When we mentally rehearse an action—making a dry run of a talk we have to give, or envisioning the fine points of our golf swing—the same neurons activate in the premotor cortex as if we had uttered those words or made that swing. Simulating an act is, in the brain, the same as performing it, except that the actual execution is somehow blocked.*

Without a defined target the mind's energy can be wasted. Many athletes have found visualization indispensable in honing their muscular skills. Imagining something in your mind's eye is essentially the same as perceiving it in the external world. It's exactly what Sally's father helped her use to ride her bicycle successfully. Imagine yourself sucking on a lemon and most likely your salivary glands respond as if you were really doing that.

The right hemisphere is strengthened through active mental picturing. When you also engage the left hemisphere with verbal language-based affirmations, the integration between the two cerebral hemispheres is enhanced.

Positive visualization may actually be used successfully to help combat old patterns of negative thinking and a negative mindset. You create pictures in your mind all the time anyway; you may as well choose to make them positive and empowering.

In *Timeless Healing: the Power and Biology of Belief,* authors Benson and Stark provided some suggestions.

> *Picture positive visual images in the mind's eye, and repeat affirmations aloud after using the Relaxation Response or Quieting Reflex* (refer to Key Factor #15). *This can be especially helpful if the brain is accustomed to ponder negative thoughts or self-criticisms.*

Actual and Virtual Rehearsal

There are two main types of rehearsal: actual and virtual. You use actual rehearsal when you participate in a cruise ship's life-boat drill or when you practice a musical instrument.

You use virtual rehearsal when you watch a video drill on an airplane or internally picture yourself practicing a musical instrument.

PET (Positron Emission Tomography) Scans have shown that in terms of recorded activity patterns in the brain, it didn't matter whether the experience was actual or virtual—the subconscious recognizes little differences between actual and virtual rehearsal. Both forms are useful and can be effective.

Motor Skills Connection

Mental practice using visualization has been shown to be effective in improving motor skills. Utilize visual and mental rehearsal, as well as physical rehearsal, in preparation for an event. Close your eyes and internally simulate the performance in your mind. Accompany this visualization with approximate physical movements. Even watching yourself doing a new behavior in your mind's eye can speed learning.

Researchers set up a study whereby an individual would practice a specific piece of music on the piano for two hours a day for seven days. At the end of the seven days, a brain scan showed that the brain's motor cortex had reshaped itself based on the fourteen hours of musical practice. Researchers then asked an equally trained individual to simply spend two hours a day for seven days imagining and picturing playing the piece of music on the piano. Practicing in your mind's eye, if you will. At the end of seven days, a brain scan showed similar reshaping of the brain's motor cortex.

One Percent Advantage Study

Researchers studied three groups of evenly matched basketball players to assess the benefits of virtual mental rehearsal versus actual real-time rehearsal. Each player was tested for accuracy in shooting baskets and a group average score was recorded. Each group of players were then given different instructions in relation to the practice of shooting baskets and tested at the end of three weeks. The results of the One Percent Advantage Study, as it came to be known, were startling.

- Players in Group One were told to refrain from any actual or virtual rehearsal related to basketball. Outcome: a zero percent change in accuracy.

- Group Two players were instructed to spend one hour per day in actual hands-on practice shooting baskets. Outcome: a 24 percent increase in accuracy.

- The players in Group Three were told to spend one hour per day in virtual mental rehearsal (internal mental picturing) with no hands-on rehearsing. Outcome: a 23 percent increase in accuracy.

There was only a one percent difference in the increase in accuracy between the group who actually practiced shooting baskets each day and those who engaged in virtual (mental) rehearsal only.

In a Cleveland Clinic Foundation study, a team of thirty healthy young adults were instructed to imagine moving the muscle of their little finger for five minutes a day, five days a week, for twelve weeks. Compared to a no-exercise control group, study participants increased their pinky-muscle strength by thirty-five percent.

Richard B. Ross put it this way:

When you engage in positive self-talk, you learn to think like an optimist. As an optimist you will be able to visualize more options and solutions to your problems. Your problem solving abilities will improve. As an optimist you will be less prone to giving into defeat.

Remembered Wellness

The term *placebo effect* is typically used to describe situations where anywhere from thirty-five to seventy percent (depending on the study) of the positive effects of a treatment or event is believed due to the person's belief in or strong expectation about what will occur. For example:

- When people walk across live coals without experiencing burns
- When allergies or cold symptoms temporarily disappear when the person wants to do something that requires the absence of symptoms
- When an individual evidences almost super-human strength in an effort to save a loved one from accident or certain death.

Dr. Herbert Benson coined new terminology for the placebo effect—*Remembered Wellness*—believing it to more accurately describe the brain functions involved when affirmative beliefs positively impact the brain-body connection. The brain is designed to think in pictures. Use visualization, internal mental picturing, regularly and by design. Mentally picture desirable behaviors and positive outcomes on a consistent basis to help you achieve your goals. Reap the benefits to your brain, your body, your health, and your potential longevity. You are the only person, however, who can do this for you.

The sixth key factor is ***Essential Exercise,*** critical for both brain and body health but misunderstood by many. The next chapter is waiting for you. Turn the page and dig in.

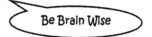

Be Brain Wise

Physical activity and exercise are critical for both your brain and body. Engage in thirty minutes of aerobic exercise at least five or six days a week. If it works better for you, break up your exercise into three ten-minute or two fifteen-minute periods of time.

For a well-rounded exercise program, include some aerobic, balance, flexibility, stretching, and resistance activities.

Key Factor—6
Essential Exercise

Exercise is the single most powerful tool you have to optimize your brain function.

—Richard Restak MD

 "Here's the bottom line, Doc," said Jock. "I don't *like* to exercise. Never have, never will. I *do* like to eat. A lot. Always have, always will. Just give me my high-blood-pressure medication and let it go at that."

"I was under the impression that you have just gotten married," said the Doctor, thoughtfully.

"I have," said Jock. "Classiest woman you ever saw. I waited until I was nearly forty to find the right one. We had a fabulous wedding and just returned from our honeymoon."

The Doctor handed Jock a flexible tape measure. "Do me a favor and measure your waist."

The tape measure would not reach all the way around Jock's waist. "Hmm-m," he murmured. "I'd guesstimate roughly 44 inches (112 centimeters). And your point would be?"

"It should be 40 inches (101 centimeters)—or less," said the Doctor. Jock shrugged rather nonchalantly.

"Listen carefully, Jock," the doctor continued, seriously. "As you may know, testosterone plays a vital role in how the body balances glucose, insulin, and fat metabolism. Studies have shown a correlation between belly fat and lowered levels of testosterone. A 2008 epidemiological study of 1,822 men by the New England Research Institutes (NERI) concluded that a man's waist circumference is the single strongest predictor of low testosterone levels. Evidence developed over the past few years now shows that, while obesity does cause low testosterone, low testosterone causes obesity. That's nothing a bridegroom wants.

"In addition, a larger waist measurement has been found to increase one's risk for diabetes type 2, asthma, and some forms of heart disease and cancer. People with high amounts of belly fat are more than three times as likely to develop memory loss and dementia later in life. You may want to rethink a healthier lifestyle in light of this research."

"What should the waist measurement be for a woman?" asked Jock.

"Generally it should be 35 inches (89 centimeters)—or less," replied the Doctor.

"Well, that puts Emily in good shape. Me? Not so much," said Jock, ruefully. "You know, Doc, I may have been a bit hasty in my comments when I arrived here today. My wife— I like the sound of that—has been suggesting we moderate our style of eating. I told her I liked her cooking and to keep it up. She's also been asking me to walk with her when we get home from work. I've put her off. Repeatedly. Tonight I'm walking and we'll be talking about meals. Thanks."

Exercise and the Brain

Many people think of physical exercise primarily in relation to their body and musculature. But physical exercise is definitely about your brain, too. Dr. Kenneth Guiffre in *The Care and Feeding of Your Brain* indicated that physical exercise helps the brain to 'boot up' efficiently, much as you would boot up a computer.

Your brain has no muscle tissue per se. Physical exercise enhances blood flow to the brain. This not only brings increased amounts of oxygen, glucose, and nutrition to brain tissues but also releases and washes away toxins and waste substances that have accumulated in the brain. Because of this, exercise has been called a general antioxidant. Studies of retirees who exercised on a regular basis showed they maintained nearly the same level of blood flow in the brain after four years, while those who chose not to exercise had a significant decrease in blood flow.

Any physical exercise can improve your brain's performance and help protect against cognitive decline. Individuals who are aerobically fit may actually have an intellectual edge. Physical exercise has been shown to improve creativity, concentration, and problem-solving. It prepares your neurons to connect, while mental stimulation allows your brain to capitalize on that readiness.

Studies of men and women over age 65 found that those who exercised were less likely to lose their mental abilities or develop dementia. But start now. In *The Owner's Manual for the Brain*, Dr. Pierce J. Howard points out that benefits are associated with *long-term* exercise.

Jennie Brand-Miller pointed out in *The New Glucose Revolution for Diabetes* that there are really only two requirements when it comes to exercise: one is that you do it; the other is that you continue to do it.

Even Plato was on the proverbial band wagon. He has been quoted as saying: Lack of activity destroys the good condition of every human being, while movement and methodical physical exercise save it and preserve it.

Ratey and Hagerman in their book *Spark: The Revolutionary New Science of Exercise and the Brain,* provide many examples of the benefits of physical exercise. Here are a few.

1. Strengthens your cardiovascular system
2. Helps to regulate glucose and insulin
3. Helps to fight obesity
4. Combats stress by dissipating cortisol
5. Improves your mood
6. Boosts your immune system
7. Strengthens your bones
8. Boosts motivation
9. Fosters neuroplasticity

Physical exercise is one way to burn off stress and boost endorphins, but the real reason it feels so good is because the brain tends to function at its best when the body gets sufficient exercise—when the heart is pumping hard and circulating the blood through your brain.

When neurons are worn down from cellular stress, synapses in the brain tend to atrophy, which eventually can sever connections between neurons. At some level your brain tries to compensate by rerouting information. But if synaptic decay outpaces the new construction, you may start noticing problems with mental, physical, or emotional function.

Many people have no idea how closely physical activity is tied to brain function. Candace B. Pert PhD pointed this out in her book *Your Body is Your Subconscious Mind*:

> *The most important function of exercise is to stimulate and cleanse the bodymind so that it is free to do its best work. You can enhance the benefits of your daily exercise by linking it to something you enjoy, such as listening to your favorite music on headphones while walking.*

And in her book *Molecules of Emotion,* Pert indicated that twenty minutes of mild aerobic exercise at the beginning of the day can turn on fat-burning neuropeptides, the effects of which can last for hours. Get up half an hour earlier. Twenty minutes is a deal for hours of fat-burning benefits.

The lifestyle you choose can accelerate or help to slow down the development of many of the symptoms typically associated with growing older. A balanced high-level-healthiness lifestyle, developed and lived in an informed manner, can not only impact the rate at which symptoms of aging crop up—at least to some degree—but help you grow older more gracefully. It can decrease your risk for heart disease, vascular disease, and diabetes.

Lifestyle also influences the mental hazards that can come with aging. The same factors that kill the body kill the brain. Dr. Mark Mattson, author of *Diet-Brain Connections,* said:

> *I think the good news—if we take it seriously—is that many of the same factors that can reduce our risk for cardiovascular disease and diabetes also reduce the risk for age-related neurodegenerative disorders.*

Dopamine and Endorphins

Physical exercise stimulates the release of dopamine, the *feel better* brain chemical that is linked with the brain's reward and pain-pleasure systems. Levels of this critical neurotransmitter tend to decrease with age so physical exercise becomes even more vital. Exercise also triggers the release of endorphins, the brain's natural morphine. Apathy is sometimes seen in the elderly, especially when they are facing the need to move into a retirement community or into an assisted living center. Regular physical exercise can help to combat apathy through the release of both dopamine and endorphins.

Inactivity, along with poor nutrition and smoking, are proven root causes of diseases. So get moving! For every hour of sitting, get up and do at least two minutes of vigorous exercise. Researchers led by Jacquelyn Kulinski MD, cardiologist, examined data from 2031 participants in the *Dallas Heart Study* ages twenty to seventy-six. They found that sitting for too long doubles the risk of diabetes. The health consequences of being too sedentary may differ from those of not getting enough physical exercise.

According to Kulinski, reducing one's daily sitting time by even one or two hours potentially could have a significant, positive impact on future cardiovascular health.

In summary: engage in physical exercise on a regular basis to increase dopamine and endorphin levels, protect your brain cells against stress, improve your mood, age-proof your brain against mental decline, and decrease your risk for heart disease, vascular disease, and diabetes. And when you reach your optimum weight-range, exercise can help you maintain it, as well.

Bottom line? You have nothing to lose and everything to gain. Get fit and then challenge yourself. If you get into shape physically, generally your mind will follow. In order to have a well-rounded exercise program, consider including: balance and flexibility activities to strengthen cerebellum function; stretching and resistance exercises to improve muscle tone.

As a reminder, consult with your physician or healthcare professional before you embark on an exercise program, especially if you have led a relatively sedentary lifestyle.

The next key factor is ***Breathing for Life.*** Take a deep breath, turn the page, and find out the reason that effective breathing is so critical for age-proofing your brain.

Be Brain Wise

Oxygen is your most essential nutrient. Brain breathe first thing in the morning to help boot up your brain. Brain breathe several more times throughout the day to increase oxygen levels in your brain.

Strive to inhale clean, fresh air. Minimize breathing polluted air whenever possible (e.g., vehicle exhaust, factory emissions, side-stream smoke).

Key Factor—7
Breath of Life

Insufficient oxygen means insufficient biological energy that can result in anything from mild fatigue to life threatening disease.

—Dr. W. Spencer Way

"Our teacher said oxygen was the body's most vital *nutrient*. That's the first time I ever heard anyone call oxygen a nutrient," said Timothy.

His father considered this for a moment. "Well," he said, "you can go without food for weeks and without water for days—but without oxygen for only a few minutes. In that sense, your teacher is probably correct."

"I'm tall for my age," said Timothy. "It's easy to slump so I don't tower over everyone. Then I breathe too shallowly."

"You got your growth spurt early," agreed his father. "However, when your classmates catch up with you, I doubt you'll want to be shorter simply because you slumped. It's one thing to breathe to stay alive. It's quite another to do effective diaphragmatic breathing that can really oxygenate your brain and body tissues and impact your athletic success positively. Think of oxygen as the breath of life."

Timothy smiled, stood tall, and breathed deeply. His father smiled back.

The Fifth Vital Sign

Your brain needs a constant supply of oxygen in order to live and function effectively. Just watch someone with emphysema struggling desperately to move air in and out of their lungs and you'll soon get the picture if you don't have it already. Oxygen from the air that moves from your lungs into the blood stream is the only way your brain gets oxygen. When you visit your doctor's office, an attendant typically takes your vital signs such as your heart rate, blood pressure, breathing rate, and body temperature. The attendant may also clip a pulse oximeter on your finger to give the doctor a general idea of how much oxygen is in your blood and how well your blood cells are saturated with oxygen. If saturation levels fall too low, it can impact brain function and health negatively. This is so important that it is often referred to as the fifth vital sign.

- Your brain uses more oxygen than any other organ in the body and about three times as much as do body muscles.

- Although your brain accounts for only two percent of your total body weight, it uses more than twenty percent of your available oxygen supply, which comes to it through circulating blood.

- The brain is filled with neurons that generally do not divide and multiply as do other cells in the body. Neurons are very sensitive to decreases in oxygen levels. They neither work very well nor survive very long without an adequate supply of oxygen.

Oxygen

As you know, oxygen is extracted from the air you breathe into your lungs, and is then transported to your brain and body through the blood stream. On average, about eight gallons of blood flow through your brain per hour delivering this vital nutrient with the help of red blood cells. As you age, your body loses some of its ability to utilize oxygen efficiently, perhaps at the rate of one percent per year from about age twenty onward.

Doctors Friedman and Martin, authors of *The Longevity Project,* point out that conscientious individuals who tend to stay healthier and live longer are less likely to smoke because smoking can decrease the relative amount of oxygen available in their lungs. If you smoke, stop. If you don't smoke, never start. Do your best to avoid breathing in sidestream smoke, polluted air, and vehicle exhaust.

According to Professor Andrew Scholey, Director of the Human Cognitive Neuroscience Unit at the University of Northumbria, extra oxygen can enhance mental performance and agility in healthy active adults. It can also ease your nerves, calm you down, and assist you in managing stressors. A report from Harvard Medical School entitled 'Boosting Your Energy' included this statement:

> *Every breath you take converts to energy. Human cells use nutrients from food and oxygen to create Adenosine Tri-Phosphate or ATP, the energy source that fuels cell function. If your cells receive too little oxygen they produce less energy.*

Benefits of Breathing

"It helps me stay alive," you say. Definitely. But there are a myriad benefits for health and longevity beyond that big one.

- Your respiratory system was designed to release as much as seventy percent of toxins through breathing. Carbon dioxide, for example. When you exhale you release carbon dioxide—a natural waste product of metabolism—that has been passed through from your bloodstream into your lungs. If you fail to breathe effectively, you may not be ridding yourself toxins, requiring other body systems to work harder, which could eventually lead to illness.

- When you inhale air your diaphragm descends and your abdomen expands. This helps massage vital organs such as the stomach, small intestine, liver and pancreas, increasing circulation. When you inhale, the upper movement of the diaphragm massages the heart. Controlled breathing can strengthen and tone your abdominal muscles, as well.

Brain Breathing

"I know how to breathe!" Of course you do. Whether or not you are breathing *effectively* is another matter altogether. Optimum breathing means you breathe deeply into your abdomen not just your chest. Even in Greek and Roman times the doctors recommended deep breathing, the voluntary holding of air in the lungs, believing that this exercise cleansed the system of impurities and gave the individuals strength.

Breathing should be deep, slow, rhythmic, and through the nose, not through the mouth. The most important part of deep breathing has to do with regulating your breaths three to four seconds in and three to four seconds out.

As a child were you told to stand straight, stick out your chest, and hold your abdomen in? Unfortunately, this represents a suboptimal position for getting air deeply into your lungs. Instead, learn to breathe using your abdominal muscles and your diaphragm. And then work to increase your lung capacity.

Brain Breathing is a specific technique to help increase the amount of oxygen that reaches your brain. Start the day with it. Aim to brain breathe several times throughout the day to ensure that high levels of oxygen infuse your brain. Here is the formula:

- Breathe in through your nose for a count of four
- Hold your breath for a count of twelve
- Exhale through pursed lips for a count of eight

Always breathe through your nose rather than your mouth if at all possible. In *Your Jaws—Your Life,* David C. Page, pointed out that breathing through your nose stimulates the release of nitric oxide, which enhances mental activity.

Peptides are brain substances composed of amino acids that impact mood. By holding your breath briefly or by breathing extra fast for several breaths, you can produce changes in the type and quantity of these peptides— and thus impact your mood.

This causes them to diffuse rapidly through your cerebrospinal fluid, which can help to elevate your mood and enhance learning. Some of these peptides are endorphins, the brain's natural morphine, so you may even reduce aches and pains. According to Candace B. Pert PhD, the peptide-respiratory link is well documented. Most peptides can be found in the respiratory center, providing the rationale for the powerful healing effects of consciously controlled breathing patterns.

You can use breathing patterns to help you learn more easily, as well. Try alternating breathing from one nostril to the other to achieve changes in short-term hemispheric processing. For example: if you are doing a left hemisphere activity, breathe through the right nostril to stimulate the left cerebral hemisphere and vice versa. If you want to alter an unwanted state, breathe through the more congested nostril.

Oxygen Deprivation

According to Nancy Zi, author of *The Art of Breathing,* incorrect breathing can contribute to vocal strain, tension, exhaustion, interfere with athletic activity and increase your risk for aches and illnesses. Shallow breathing leads to less air in the lungs, reducing oxygen transfer into the blood 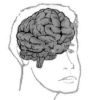 stream, and potentially resulting in devastating consequences for brain function. Insufficient oxygen to the brain can contribute to mental sluggishness, negative thoughts, sleep apnea, poor concentration, forgetfulness, mood swings, restlessness, depressive thoughts, decreased alertness, and problems with memory functions and judgment.

Vision and hearing may decline. Lack of adequate oxygen is now believed to be a contributor to heart disease, stroke, cancer, and fatigue—one of the most common problems experienced by people worldwide. Other conditions may contribute to a potential reduction in blood-oxygen levels, as well: asthma, emphysema, chronic stress, air pollution, traveling at high elevation, clogged arteries, and a sedentary life style,

Yawning

Did you grow up being told that when people yawned in a meeting or classroom that it meant they were bored? Those may be triggers but researchers now suggest that sleep-deprivation may also trigger yawning. The temperature of your brain increases when you are sleep deprived. The involuntary behavior of yawning (it's difficult to produce a genuine yawn on demand) may be designed to cool down brain tissue.

Yawning causes you to take in deeper breaths of air. Inhaling cool air ventilates your sinuses and helps to dissipate heat. This is another way in which human brains resemble computers: computers and human brains work best when cool. Good breathing techniques used consciously, by design, can help you both oxygenate and cool brain and body tissues. Adequate amounts of oxygen are essential for optimum brain and body function. Breathe—for your life.

Key factor number eight involves the vital importance of avoiding dehydration. The next chapter is waiting for you— as soon as you grab a drink of water.

Be Brain Wise

Avoid dehydration like the proverbial plague. It can contribute to a variety of undesirable conditions from wrinkles in your skin to an increased risk of blood clots and shrinkage of brain tissue.

Minimize the likelihood of your body reabsorbing waste products through your skin by keeping it clean. Reduce your risk of being a pee brain by drinking enough water each day to achieve a couple of pale urines.

Key Factor—8
Wonderful Water

The water cycle and the life cycle are one.

—Jacques Cousteau

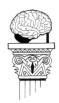 "This seminar is really interesting," said Sally to her husband after the morning break. "I'm so glad we decided to attend." Colin nodded. "I knew about the importance of changing your clothing frequently and bathing to wash away impurities that are released through the skin, but I didn't quite realize the importance of water internally." The couple Sally resumed their seats.

"This business of dehydration is serious," the speaker said beginning the next section. "Some reports estimate that the brain is at least three-fourths water and may have a higher percentage of water than any other body organ—if it is properly hydrated. Your body is sixty or seventy percent fluid. Both brain and body need a daily supply of pure water to do their jobs well. And if you fail to give it the amount of water it needs on a daily basis, get ready for problems."

"Maybe we need to look at this more carefully," Colin whispered, turning to Sally. "I doubt either one of us drinks enough water. I'm sure I don't."

"We mostly drink fruit juice and coffee at breakfast and soft drinks the rest of the day," agreed Sally, whispering back.

The speaker continued. "If you don't drink enough water, your brain will have to find another source. It will direct the body to steal some fluid from elsewhere in your body. At any given time your bladder has the largest potential reservoir of fluid anywhere in your body—urine. If the brain gets desperate for fluid, it may instruct the body to concentrate the urine in your bladder, trying to obtain some additional liquid—which it can then send up to the brain." The speaker paused rather dramatically. "In my book, that puts a different spin on the term *pee* brain."

Sally and Colin both burst out laughing. "I've never heard of that before," said Sally, "and it's not a pleasant thought!"

"Me either," said Colin. "But I can tell you one thing, I'll remember it. *Pee brain* indeed—not on my watch!"

Water is the most important essential for life. Your brain and body need water to live. Period. You can get along without food for longer than you can survive without water. As one writer put it, perhaps tongue-in-cheek, millions of people have lived without love—not one has lived without water.

A vital nutrient that must be supplied from an outside source, water is also the most neglected in many people's lives. As Linda Boeckner and Kay McKinzie point out in their article 'Water: The Nutrient:' *'Water deprivation kills faster than the lack of any other nutrient.'*

According to Neil Nedley MD, author of *Proof Positive, a* lack of water causes dehydration of red blood cells, making them less flexible, and they have a greater tendency to clot.

A Global Drinking Problem

A common *drinking problem* around the world involves a failure to drink enough water. This can lead to chronic dehydration, a major contributor to headaches. Symptoms of dehydration can include dry mouth, dry skin, sense of thirst, sleepiness, headache, decreased urine output, and constipation. Dehydration can lead to lethargy, impaired learning, and an increased risk for stroke and heart disease,

 Has your brain been locked away from a daily supply of pure water? Keeping your brain well hydrated can help avoid shrinkage of brain tissue, a condition that has been linked with memory problems and Alzheimer's. Dehydration increases the production of damaged molecules known as free radicals, which also have been associated with a higher risk of developing symptoms of dementia later on in life and can wreak havoc in many ways.

In her article 'Dehydration in the Elderly: A Short Review,' Risa J. Lavizzo-Mourey pointed out that dehydration is the most common fluid and electrolyte problem among the elderly. The rate of aging and one's level of water consumption appear to be directly related—dehydration can contribute to premature aging. Water is absolutely essential for avoiding dehydration and yet many are chronically dehydrated. One contributor may be that many drink water only when they are thirsty and by then the brain and body are likely already dehydrated. In addition, with advancing age, most people tend to lose some of their thirst sensations. With diminished thirst awareness they don't even realize their brain and body need water.

Another contributor—as Candace B. Pert PhD, author of *Molecules of Emotion* pointed out—is that the sensations for hunger and thirst are quite similar and easily confused; a confusion that often begins during early childhood. Parents often feed babies when they are thirsty, instead of giving them water to drink. This means that growing up and in adulthood many eat because they think they are hungry when actually they're thirsty. When you mistake thirst for hunger you may be tempted to overeat or drink some food (e.g., milk, fruit juices, and shakes) or down unhealthy snacks. Ingesting extra calories from foods and beverages, rather than giving your brain and body the water they need, can have implications beyond dehydration: an exhausted digestive system, weight gain, and so on.

According to Dr. Mu Shik Jhon, author of *The Water Puzzle and the Hexagonal Key,* outward signs of growing older, such as wrinkling and withering, reflect what is happening inside the body. At the cellular level, growing older can cause a shift in the ratio of water inside versus outside the cells, because the body's water content tends to decrease with age. As the volume of water inside the cells is reduced, the cells *wither.* Jhon believes that water is the perfect means of energy transfer within biological systems, since water has the capacity to hold so much energy.

In his book *Your Body's Many Cries for Water* Fereydoon Batmanghelidjh MD explains that water is the body's main source of energy. Water flows through cell membranes providing electrical energy much like turbines in a hydroelectric plant. A lack of water is one of the most common causes of daytime fatigue.

Water before Each Meal

In his book *Hexagonal Water - The Ultimate Solution,* author M. J. Pangman recommends drinking a glass of water twenty or thirty minutes before each meal. This not only helps to prevent dehydration but also helps the body learn to distinguish between thirst and hunger. This is important for those who are trying to maintain optimum weight since the average person tends to eat slightly less at a meal when they drink a glass of water first. This means that drinking water before a meal not only helps with hydration but may also reduce one's caloric intake at the next meal.

Researcher L. Van Welleghen and colleagues studied water preloading before eating. The results showed a significantly lower caloric intake for the older group of participants. Interestingly enough, water preloading did not show a significantly lower caloric intake for the younger group of study participants (ages twenty-one to thirty-five) but it did help with their overall hydration.

When you prevent dehydration through appropriate water intake, you may find it easier to maintain your optimum weight. Pay attention and earn to differentiate between thirst and hunger. If you sense 'hunger pangs,' especially if it is not mealtime, drink a glass of water and reevaluate your hunger in thirty minutes or so. How long has it been since you had a nutritious meal? What are your energy-expenditure patterns for the last few hours? Does your brain and body need water? If your hunger pangs signal that your brain and body really need food for energy, by all means eat. Otherwise, drink water.

Diet-Drink Myth

Some people rarely drink water, per se. Instead they have developed the habit of drinking fruit juices, punch, tea, coffee, hot chocolate, soda drinks, alcohol, or any number of other types of beverages when thirsty. Perhaps even worse, many choose diet drinks on a regular basis because they believe it will help them to lose weight—or at least prevent them from gaining. Wrong! Diet drinks can sabotage your high-level-healthiness lifestyle. This is because diet drinks tend to stimulate the release of insulin, which typically results in a blood sugar low. The upshot from the blood sugar low is that the individuals are prompted to increase the number of calories ingested the next time they eat, which increases their risk for obesity. Avoid diet drinks like the proverbial plague.

Drink Beyond Thirst

Eight glasses of water per day has long been touted as the needed amount. Information from the Mayo Clinic, as reported in the Sept/Oct 2000 issue of *Vibrant Life,* has gone a long way to revise this recommendation. Researchers found that the average male who metabolizes about 2,900 calories a day may need at least 96 ounces (2.8 liters) of water, while a woman who burns 2,200 calories a day may need at least 72 ounces (2.1 liters) of water.

If the weather is very hot and you are exercising, doing heavy muscular work, and/or perspiring, you may need to drink even more to replace the amount that has been lost. And proportionally, children may need to drink not only more water but also more frequently than adults.

Rather than trying to count glasses of water, James Peters MD, Medical Director at the St. Helena Center for Health, recommends simply adjusting the amount of water you drink each day based on the color of your urine. Drink enough water to achieve two clear or very pale urines per day. If you have been drinking less water than your brain and body need, be aware that as you increase your water intake you may also increase your visits to the toilet—initially. As your brain and body begin to trust that you are going to provide them with sufficient water on a daily basis, your bladder will usually adjust as well. (Be sure to talk with your physician if you have a medical condition that requires reduced water intake.) Remember that you lose approximately one pint (16 ounces or 0.4 liters) of water each day just from exhaling air from your lungs—all of which must be replaced!

Bottom line? Make pure water your primary beverage and choose to love drinking it. Water does not activate your digestive system in the way that drinking juice or soft drinks or sugary beverages do. Water hydrates brain and body, lowers your risk of dehydration, and gives your digestive system a rest.

Pure water has no taste, no color, and no odor. It can't really even be defined easily but it is necessary to life itself. According to Antoine de Saint-Exupery, author of the famous book *The Little Prince,* individuals who primarily drink beverages other than water miss something because water "fills us with a gratification that exceeds the delight of the senses." Water is the beverage of champions!

Are you hungry? Key factor nine is ***Macronutrition Medley.*** Turn the page. It's waiting for you.

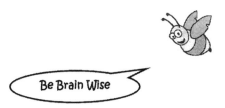

Be Brain Wise

Plan meals on a regular basis for your brain's sake. Select a variety of nutritious and primarily plant-based foods: fruits, grains, nuts, and vegetables that contain vital macronutrients to power your brain and body. Eat them in as natural a state as possible.

Choose carefully what you ingest—and where and when and how—as if your life depends upon it. Because it does!

Key Factor—9
Macronutrition Medley

*Put good food into your brain each day—
you are what you eat.*

—Daniel G. Amen MD

 Andy parked his bright red sports car—a 'mid-life-crisis' purchase—in front of his friend's auto mechanic shop and got out. "Hey. Andy," said Billy-Bob. "What did Doc say about your cough? Are you on your death bed or do you get to hang around for a while longer?"

Andy grimaced. "My walking-pneumonia is back and Doc nearly put me in the hospital. Said all the fast food calories I chow down are not only increasing my weight but also suppressing my immune system. I asked him what a calorie was and he told me it's the name for a unit of energy—but that not all calories are created equal." Andy took a sheet of paper from his pocket. "I'm supposed to stop eating *white* sugar, flour, rice, and pasta; refined and processed products made with them, fried foods, trans fats, and hydrogenated or partially hydrogenated oils. What's left?"

"Probably high quality fruits, nuts, grains, and veggies," replied Billy-Bob, "in as natural a state as possible. I know what you eat: fast, fried, fat, and frozen, washed down with sodas and topped with as many desserts as you can hold. Really, Andy, were the Doctor's comments a surprise?"

Seeing Andy start to bristle, Billy-Bo added quickly: "Hey, pal, you know I'm on your side but this is your third bout with pneumonia this year. People die from pneumonia! You wouldn't put poor quality low-octane fuel in that red beauty out front. You're much more valuable than it is and yet you subsist on low quality junk food. Go figure."

"I know," said Andy, frowning. "The Doc made me an appointment with a nutritional coach who can help me move to a healthier plant-based diet, which, the doctor said, just might save my life. Okay. I'm not ready to cash it in yet. I can learn—and change." The two friends high-fived.

Macronutrients refer to foods that provide nutrition in the form of calories. High quality macronutrients include unrefined, unprocessed foods (fruits, grains, seeds, nuts, vegetables) in as natural a state as possible along with healthier plant fats. Your brain and body are nourished by high-quality nutrition. Less desirable foods are usually dense, refined and processed, and of lower quality. Often dubbed 'empty' calories, they can add weight to your frame but contribute little if any quality nutrition. It's really pretty simple. Ingest 3,500 calories more than you use and add one pound to your weight. Expend 3,500 more calories than you take in and you stand to lose a pound.

The quality of your macronutrition affects your neurochemistry, which in turn influences your brain, mood, actions and behaviors, thought processes, and even emotions and feelings. Macronutrients are typically grouped into three general categories: carbohydrates, fats, and proteins.

Carbohydrates: Carbs contribute four calories per gram. According to Elisa Zied RD, carbs are not the enemy. Donald Layman PhD, professor of human nutrition at the University of Illinois, has said: "Carbohydrates are the only nutrients that exist solely to fuel the body." They are used easily for energy by all cells and tissues and can be stored in muscles and the liver for use later on. They are needed for the brain and Central Nervous System or CNS, kidneys, and muscles—including those of the heart—to function properly. Like calories, however, as Andy's doctor pointed out, carbs are not all created equal. Frank Sacks MD, nutrition professor at the Harvard T.H. Chan School of Public Health, has said that the quality of your carbs is as important as the quantity. Carbs can be divided into three groups: simple, complex, and fiber.

1. Simple carbs contain one or two sugars and digest quite quickly. Fructose, for example. It is found in whole fruits that also contribute valuable vitamins and other nutrients. On the other hand, high fructose corn syrup, metabolized in the liver, can spike blood sugar levels and trigger weight gain. Eating too many refined and processed simple carbs (e.g., white rice, white flour, and white sugar) can lead to an increase in total calories ingested and to an increased risk of obesity.

2. Complex carbohydrates contain three or more sugars that not only digest more slowly but also deliver fiber and valuable vitamins and minerals. Healthier carbs include steel-cut oats and rye, brown rice, quinoa, buckwheat, millet, whole-grain barley, seeds, legumes such as beans and lentils, beets, and starchy vegetables such as yams.

3. Fiber is key for gastrointestinal health and the timely and appropriate elimination of waste. Fiber can be divided into soluble and insoluble forms. Soluble fiber absorbs liquid and forms a gel, which can help resolve diarrhea by removing excess fluid from the bowel. It can help lower blood cholesterol and glucose levels. Examples includes: strawberries, blueberries, apples, avocado, dried figs and prunes, oranges, and mangos; asparagus, edamame, broccoli, green beans and peas, carrots, legumes, oats, barley, and peanuts. Insoluble fiber passes through the intestines largely intact, increasing stool bulk, which can help resolve constipation. Whole grains top the list of insoluble fiber along with air-popped popcorn, zucchini, broccoli, cabbage, leafy greens, and root vegetables; plus most beans and legumes, raspberries, unpeeled apples and grapes, walnuts, almonds, and sunflower seeds.

Prebiotics are types of carbohydrates that are resistant to digestion in humans. They reach the colon intact where they selectively feed many strains of beneficial bacteria. Resistant Starch or RS is one type of prebiotic and is being touted as protective against colorectal cancer. RS is found in seeds, for example, and legumes such as lentils and some other beans, bananas, and partially milled grains. That's the reason some prefer sourdough bread made with coarse rye or cracked multi-grains and seeds for the prebiotic resistant starch it contains.

Dietary guidelines issued by the United States Department of Agriculture (USDA) recommend that forty-five to sixty-five percent of one's total calories come from carbs, preferably from healthier high-quality sources, of course.

Andrew Weil MD has said that it is important to eat some carbohydrates at breakfast because the brain needs to boot up in the morning after the 'fast' during sleep, and it does that best with carbs. Preferably healthier carbs, of course. The mitochondria, tiny factories within cells, convert oxygen and other nutrients into adenosine triphosphate or ATP, the chemical energy that powers metabolic processes. The mitochondria convert carbohydrates into glucose, fuel for brain and body. The brain consumes a quarter pound of glucose per day—more glucose (fuel) than any other organ in the body except for muscles used during heavy physical exercise.

According to Benjamin V. Treadwell MD, most glucose in the body is used to manufacture neurotransmitters, the substances needed to propagate electro-chemical signals via the electrical circuitry of the nervous system. If insufficient glucose is available due to dieting or low quality foods, other tissues will decrease their consumption of glucose and of Vitamin B7 or biotin (also needed to manufacture neurotransmitters) in an attempt to allow a greater supply for the brain. There is some concern regarding the potential long-term impact of 'low-carb diets' on the optimum functioning of the brain and nervous system. Foods that are believed to strengthen brain function include blueberries, broccoli, beans, oats, oranges, spinach, soy, tomatoes, wild salmon, walnuts, and yogurt. Studies by Bell and Martin at the University of Reading in the UK found that blueberry flavonoids are linked with memory and learning. An article by Mary Franz in the January 2011 Scientific American MIND, reported that compounds common to berries, tofu, tea, and other foods can shore up memory and boost brainpower.

Fats: Fats contribute nine calories per gram, more than twice the amount in carbohydrates or proteins—so go easy on them. Too much fat in your menu may translate into weight gain and/or an increased risk for cardiovascular diseases. It is important to eat some healthier fats as they help keep your skin and hair in good condition, assist in absorbing the so-called fat-soluble vitamins A, D, E, and K; and provide essential fatty acids. Some recommend plant-based fats such as cold-pressed olive oil for salads and coconut oil for cooking.

Myelin, the insulation around nerve axons, is about seventy percent fat. Oleic acid, one of the most common fatty acids in myelin, is found in cold-pressed olive oil as well as in almonds, pecans, macadamias, peanuts, and avocados. Structurally, brain tissue is composed of a 1:1 ratio of omega-6 to omega-3 fatty acids. A high intake of meat and dairy products may lead to a ratio of 20:1. An imbalance of fatty acids may be linked to hyperactivity, depression, some mental illnesses, and possibly some allergies.

Learn to read labels—and then take time to read them. Carry a magnifying glass, if need be. Avoid hydrogenated or partially hydrogenated oils and trans fats and minimize the use of saturated fats from animal sources. Be judicious in the amount of plant-based fats you take in on a daily basis.

Proteins: proteins contribute four calories per gram. They are large complex molecules composed of amino acids. Proteins are needed for the structure, processes, proper functioning, repair, and regulation of the organs and tissues of the human body—including the brain and nervous system.

Current Dietary Guidelines for Americans recommend that the average person should aim to get from ten to thirty-five percent of their daily calories from protein (depending on their activities). Some ingest more protein than their brain and body need, while others, often the very elderly, may not eat quite enough. The Physicians Committee for Responsible Medicine (PCRM), which includes eminent physicians Doctors Dean Ornish and John McDougall, recommends getting most of your macronutrition from plant-based vegetables, fruits, whole grains, nuts, and beans (with small amounts of animal products for those not wishing to eat vegetarian or vegan).

Pay attention to how your brain and body respond to different foods. Do your joints ache after eating nightshades (e.g., white potatoes, eggplant, tomatoes, and green peppers)? Does your brain feel foggy after eating high-sugar foods? Are you waking up with a hangover more frequently? Make brain-friendly choices. Fortunately there is a medley of quality foods from which to choose. Select natural, unrefined, and unprocessed foods with a low Glycemic Index and Glycemic Load—to avoid spiking blood sugar (glucose) levels in your brain. Take thoughtful measured steps. Even small changes can be helpful over the long term. Your brain, body, and immune system will appreciate your efforts.

Do you know how macronutrition and micronutrition differ? Turn the page for key factor number ten, *Micronutrition Mystery.*

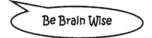

Be Brain Wise

According to Gary W. Arendash PhD, Research Professor at Florida Alzheimer's Research Center:

'In order to optimize brain function over your lifespan, high amounts of brain nutrients are required from both food and supplements.'

Consider including green superfoods in your high-level-healthiness lifestyle to strengthen immune system function and support optimum brain function.

Key Factor—10
Micronutrition Mystery

*Supplements have a profound effect on when and to what
degree your mind can boot up to full capacity.*

—Kenneth Giuffre MD, Theresa Foy DiGeronimo

"Stephen, apparently there's a new medical specialty that is researching *micronutrients*, whatever they are," said Esther, handing the newspaper to her husband. "Look at this article."

Stephen read aloud: "A new medical specialty, Nutritional Neuroscience, is studying and discovering how to keep the brain functioning at peak power for as long as possible. For some, that is an entire lifetime. Researchers are investigating ways in which micronutrients—fod factors needed by the body in small amounts such as vitamins, trace minerals, and enzymes—can be utilized to prevent and sometimes even reverse brain deterioration related to aging or neurological diseases. Advances in brain imaging and other research equipment has made it possible for scientists to track the impact of micronutritional factors on brain function."

"That's probably what Dr. Paul Clayton, Research Director of Medical Nutrition Matters in Oxford, was referring to when he said that modern lifestyles have increased the external threats to our health," Stephen added.

"Actually, I'm not surprised," said Esther, "the way food is grown, fertilized, sprayed, waxed, usually harvested unripe, shipped, stored, radiated, and you name it. By the time we bring it home from the supermarket it's amazing there is much quality nutrition left in it at all."

"Hmm-m," said Stephen, nodding. "This article also talks about something called *green superfoods*. Listen to this: 'The American Commission on Anti-Aging referred to green superfoods as the closest to a perfect food this planet can offer.' The author recommends eating some of them every day, especially as one gets older.'" Stephen paused briefly and then continued reading aloud.

"Green superfoods are a special category of micronutrient-rich foods (e.g., kelp, young cereal grasses such as wheat, kamut, barley, alfalfa, and rye). Filled with vitamins and trace minerals and containing about a third of all the known enzymes. Plus they help diminish hunger cravings. World-renowned scientist and recipient of Japan's prestigious Science and Technology Award, Yoshide Hagiwara MD, has said that young barley grass, a green superfood, is one of the most nutritionally balanced foods in nature."

"Our neighbors have planted a small garden in their side-yard," said Esther. "They got some old wine barrels, cut them in half, and filled them with potting soil. They've planted herbs along with radishes, lettuce, tomatoes, squash, and cucumbers. They're already having fun picking 'veggies' for lunch. I'm going to tell them about green superfoods. They could grow a small patch of greens— young barley grass or wheat or alfalfa—and cut some off each morning to mix in their smoothies."

"Oh," she added. "I just realized that's probably what those little trays of greens are in the juice bar at the mall."

"We can do what our neighbors are doing," said Stephen, chuckling. "We've got that old bathtub that's been sitting in the garage. We can fill it with potting soil and plant barley and wheat and alfalfa ourselves. Every morning we can cut an inch of some of the baby grasses and add it to *our* breakfast smoothies. By alternating which ones we use each day, they should keep growing and last a long time." He turned to look at his wife. Esther was already walking toward the garage.

Micronutritional Link

Micronutrients include substances that are critical to optimum brain function and vital to health, but unlike macronutrients add few, if any, calories to your daily menu. Many do not give their brain sufficient enzymes, vitamins, minerals, phytonutrients and phytochemicals, and adaptogens. Studies have shown a connection between good micronutrition and enhanced learning, memory retention, the ability to counteract stress and prevent disease. For example, B vitamins may lower high homocysteine levels, which have been associated with strokes and Alzheimer's. The reverse is also true. Inadequate micronutrition may increase your risk for illnesses and disease.

Most people are familiar with vitamins and minerals. Some even with enzymes. There are other micronutrients that are less well-known, however. Following are examples of some of these.

L-Theanine. L-Theanine is a unique non-protein amino acid that is involved in the formation of a brain chemical known as gamma amino butyric acid or GABA for short. It influences the levels of dopamine, the feel better chemical. It also impacts serotonin, connected with sleep and an ability of the brain to experience joy. L-Theanine has also been shown to improve learning ability and memory, exert protective effects on the brain by antagonizing glutamate toxicity, and stimulate the release of nerve growth factor (NGF), a protein that increases the growth of dendrites and that is needed by cholinergic brain cells that use acetylcholine for signaling. It is found in green tea and some nutritional supplements made from green tea.

Antioxidants. In *A Report from the American Commission on Anti-Aging,* Robert Concoby is quoted as saying: 'Longevity depends on the amount of antioxidant reserves left over after normal cell function has taken place.' What are they and what do they do? Most people these days have heard the term *free radical*, a damaged atom or molecule that has lost one of its paired electrons. Free radicals can accelerate the rate of aging, destroy brain cells, and hasten development of Alzheimer's disease. Free radicals can be created during cell processes within the body when something goes wrong with the creation of new cells. Free radicals can also be taken in from outside sources by breathing in polluted air, tobacco smoke, and vehicle exhaust.

Antioxidants such as Vitamin C and Vitamin E, Carotene, Beta-Carotene, Selenium, Lecithin, and Superoxide Dismutase (SOD) have been shown to neutralize free radicals.

They 'donate' electrons to replace the missing electron, which can help to prevent some of the damage free radicals can cause. Antioxidants are found in higher concentrations in some foods. For example:

- Cranberries, blueberries, and blackberries along with red, purple, and blue grapes

- Red pinto beans, kidney beans, and black beans; artichokes, russet potatoes, pumpkin and squash

- Pecans, walnuts, and hazelnuts. They rank highest in the nut category.

Fatty Acids. Fatty acids play a role in regulating blood pressure, triglyceride and cholesterol levels, and in keeping the arteries healthy. A supply of fatty acids is critical to the health of cell membranes that surround the neurons. And healthy cell membranes are required for appropriate electrical function. These important energy-supplying molecules can be broken down to provide adenosine triphosphate (ATP), the energy currency of living systems.

Lecithin is an excellent source of essential fatty acids, while flaxseed oil (the vegetable alternative to fish oil) has been found to contain omega-3 fatty acids. For those who enjoy eating fish, fatty acids are also found in some fish. Avoid deep-frying them, however. (The fish, not the people!)

Phytonutrients or Phytochemicals. These plant-derived chemical compounds are undergoing scientific research for their potential health-promoting properties. Carotenoids are probably the most well-known and the most researched.

Carotenoids have been linked to decreased risk of stroke, increased blood flow in the brain, and the repair and maintenance of neuronal structures. They are found in orange-colored fruits and vegetables such as sweet potatoes and carrots. Typically, the darker the color, the more carotenoids the foods contain. Red, purple, and blue grapes have been found to contain phytonutrients. Resveratrol, a substance believed to be good for the heart, is contained in the skin of these dark-colored grapes so avoid peeling the grapes.

Adaptogens. Adaptogenic herbs have been found to increase the body's resistance to stress and trauma while improving energy, stamina, sleep, and the overall functioning of the brain. Adaptogens found in ginseng and mushroom extract help to maintain the balance of neurotransmitters during stress (e.g., help to prevent increases in cortisol and decreases in serotonin and norepinephrine).

Different Strokes . . .

Because every brain is different, not every brain and body respond to the same nutritional product in the same way. That may or may not be a reflection of the specific nutritional product itself, but may reflect what that specific brain needed at the moment in the way of micronutrition. Because heat tends to destroy enzymes, it is important to select green superfoods that have not been prepared by heating. Ingest high quality foods in as natural a state as possible. Include green superfoods and appropriate nutritional products that can provide you with the vitamins, minerals, and enzymes that your brain and body need.

Grow herbs and young grasses in your own yard, if possible, to increase the availability of green superfoods.

Decades ago Thomas Edison predicted that the doctor of the future 'will give no medicine, but will interest patients in the care of the human frame, in a proper diet, and in the cause and prevention of disease.'

Together your brain and immune system constitute the most amazing prevention and healing system on the planet. Increase your knowledge about micronutrients and give your brain what it needs. Investigate nutritional products carefully and make selections that help you to self-medicate your brain's stew in a positive way.

Add to that the words of Albert Schweitzer MD, when he said: 'Each patient carries his own doctor inside him—we are at our best when we give the doctor who resides within a chance to go to work.'

Choose the highest quality foods possible, knowing you are providing powerful and necessary micronutrition to help support your invaluable immune system and to strengthen and preserve your brain function. Micronutrients can help to give the doctor who resides within you a chance to go to work—so you can be at your best. So you can live a lot of years with lots of life in those years.

Key factor eleven speaks to the critical desirability of maintaining an optimum weight. As with other aspects of health, wellness, and longevity, prevention tends to be easier than cure but in most cases it is possible to get one's weight within a desirable range.

Be Brain Wise

Oprah Winfrey has been reported as saying, 'Getting my lifelong weight struggle under control has come from a process of treating myself as well as I treat others in every way.'

Embrace high-level-healthiness living to help you maintain an optimum body weight and Body Mass Index (BMI) for your gender, size, and bone structure, as well as an appropriate waist circumference. Treat yourself as well as you treat others—every day and in every way.

Key Factor—11
Weighing Weight

Being obese is like being twenty years older than you really are. It does more damage to your quality of life, causes more chronic medical conditions, and incurs more healthcare expenditures than either smoking or alcohol abuse.

—Roland Sturm, RAND Corporation Economist

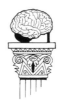 "I've tried every diet and weight-loss trick in the book," said Ellen. "Nothing works. My weight weighs on me, to say nothing of the scales. I blame my mother. While pregnant with me, she gained 90 pounds, hung onto them for the rest of her life, and added more. At her death she weighed 400 pounds."

"Blaming doesn't help," said her neighbor, chuckling. "It's just an attempt to displace some of one's own discomfort onto another person. Your mother likely did the best she could at the time with what she knew. Most people do. I've finally learned that I'm responsible for how much I weigh."

"Not true!" exclaimed Ellen. "I come by my overweight honestly. When are people going to get that *big is beautiful* and stop trying to get us to *get smaller*?"

Few topics can elicit outrage faster than questions or comments about weight. And few topics are as riddled with excuses, denial, blaming, and rationalizations.

If you've gotten stuck in the blame game, and it's easy to do, ponder this quote attributed to Steve Goodier: 'An important decision I made was to resist playing the blame game. The day I realized that I am in charge of how I will approach problems in my life, that things will turn out better or worse because of me and nobody else, that was the day I knew I would be a happier and healthier person. And that was the day I knew I could truly build a life that matters.'

Definitions

The World Health Organization or WHO defines overweight and obesity as an abnormal or excessive fat accumulation that may impair one's health. Overweight means you have a Body Mass Index or BMI greater than or equal to 25. Obesity means a BMI greater than or equal to 30.

Lugging around excess fat is not good for the brain and can lead to brain atrophy, which is linked with cognitive decline. MRI studies by Paul Thompson PhD, UCLA Professor of Neurology, revealed that brains of overweight individuals showed 4 percent less brain tissue, while obese brains had 8 percent less tissue than those of normal-weight people. The brains of overweight persons looked 8 years older and those of obese individuals looked 16 years older than those of normal-weight people.

Obesity is linked with more than 50 diseases—including type 2 diabetes, high blood pressure, cardiovascular disease, cancer and cancer reoccurrence, and dementia. Obesity may even be worse for females. Women who are obese throughout life are at increased risk for developing dementia, perhaps due to increased secretion of cortisol.

Waist Circumference

Lugging excess weight around one's middle is an especially ugly risk factor for a testosterone-estrogen hormone imbalance. Testosterone plays a vital role in how the body balances glucose and insulin and in fat metabolism in both males and females. *Aromatase*, an enzyme in fat tissue, converts testosterone into estradiol, a type of estrogen. That can result in a decrease in testosterone levels and a corresponding increase in estrogen levels, undesirable for anyone regardless of gender. Snacks or meals loaded with refined and processed carbohydrates from white flour and sugar can trigger the biggest surge in aromatase.

The New England Research Institutes (NERI) reported a study of 1,822 men, which concluded that a man's waist circumference is the single strongest predictor of low testosterone. It's a two-way street: obesity can cause low testosterone and low testosterone can contribute to obesity.

The American Cancer Society reported that researchers followed 6,885 women who were treated with standard chemotherapy for breast cancer for eight years. They found a thirty percent higher risk of cancer recurrence and a fifty percent higher risk of death for women who were overweight when compared with death rates for women of normal weight who had breast cancer.

Dieting Trap

Samuel Beckett said, 'Probably nothing in the world arouses more false hopes than the first four hours of a diet.' Those concerned about their weight can get caught in dieting traps.

That's unfortunate, since many have made their fortunes on the back of the 'diet craze,' offering seemingly endless options: crash, fast, no-carb, hi-fat, low-fat, juice, raw food, fat farms, boot camp, and so on. When one type falls out of favor, it's often brought back under a new name.

UCLA researcher Stuart Wolpert found dieting does not work. By their very nature diets are designed to fail. Initially you many lose a few pounds as the brain and body respond temporarily to something new and different. But dieting cannot be maintained over time, especially when it involves food deprivation. Within a space of just two to three years, most eventually gain back everything they lost—often more—and risk damaging brain and body systems in the process. A study published in the journal American Psychologist found that dieting does not lead to sustained weight loss or health benefits for the majority of people.

The first step in escaping a diet trap is to recognize that you are in one. Stop dieting. If you aren't dieting, don't start. Instead, adjust what you eat, when you eat, and how much you eat as part of a high-level-healthiness lifestyle—and do that for the rest of your life.

A Step at a Time

How much someone weighs—*not that it is anyone else's business, you understand*—fuels cartoons, jokes, and stand-up comedy routines. It can also trigger discouragement, depression, and illness. Although nearly two thirds of the American population are outside their ideal-weight range, many do little more than talk about it—if they do that. Health and longevity begin with respecting yourself.

Respecting yourself *enough*, that is, to take very good care of yourself. According to Researcher Lin Yang PhD, this generation of Americans is the first that may have a shorter life expectancy than the previous generation. Obesity is one of the biggest contributors, no pun intended, because it drives so many chronic health conditions and diseases.

Overweight and obesity occur an ounce at a time—so do weight loss and prevention. Eating 3,500 calories more than you expend can lead to a gain of 1 pound (454 grams). Of course the reverse is also true. Fortunately, maintaining your optimum weight does not mean going hungry. Pioneer researchers such as Doctors Dean Ornish and John McDougall have demonstrated that generally you can eat as much as you want of the foods they recommend for daily consumption—without gaining weight.

Balance *what* and *when* you eat and drink with your level of physical activity and exercise, your mindset, attitude, and self-talk, along with your over-all lifestyle choices. This is key to maintaining an optimum weight. Millions are getting on board with a longevity lifestyle worldwide.

Manage Your Expectations

Many have unrealistic expectations of what they *should* weigh. An optimum weight for you likely will have nothing to do with pictures of nearly anorexic models in magazines. It does need to match who *you* are in terms of size, shape, and bone structure, and be doable for the rest of your life. Evaluate expectations carefully and select those that are realistic and that *you* want to meet. You make daily choices that move you toward or away from your optimum weight.

It's usually not about food anyway. It's often about using food to self-medicate and to alter your neurochemistry to help you feel better. Remember: everything starts in your brain. Being either too heavy or too thin are both bad for your brain and, therefore, for your body as well.

A Few Tips

- Stay hydrated. Drink plenty of water and avoid all sodas, diet drinks, sugary drinks, and artificial sweeteners. Drink a glass of water twenty to thirty minutes before eating to make sure you are not thirsty and to dampen down Ghrelin, your brain's 'let's eat' hormone.

- Eat slowly and chew your food thoroughly. The brain typically signals it has had enough after about fifteen or twenty minutes of eating, which activates Leptin, your brain's 'I've had enough' hormone.

- Eat quality food in as natural a state as possible. Minimize the use of *white* sugar, flour, rice, pasta, and refined and processed foods made with them. Avoid trans fats and hydrogenated/partially-hydrogenated fats.

- Avoid these four food groups: *fast, fried, fat*, and *frozen*. Generally avoid snacking between meals, especially on items that trigger a blood-sugar spike to your brain.

- If you are in the midst of a difficult situation, eat lightly or wait to eat until you are in a better environment. Develop good stress-management techniques to avoid emotional eating. Manage your emotions and feelings in effective ways other than through food.

- Stay active. Get regular physical exercise. Weigh once a week. Gauge your progress by how your clothing fits.

- Move toward a Mediterranean-style plant-based cuisine, eating more fruits and veggies every day. Include some seeds and raw nuts and a variety of whole grains.

- Eat nutritious meals at regular times and reduce your caloric intake slightly as you grow older. Two meals a day may be all you need, especially if you're retired and/or do mostly sedentary work. For three meals: eat like a king for breakfast, a prince for lunch, and a pauper for your third meal. Try two bites of healthy dessert—once in a while—eaten slowly.

- Periodically keep a food journal for three to seven days. Studies have shown this strategy to be a consistently helpful tool for many and can help sleuth out what is sabotaging your success.

Do you recall the old television program (ancient, actually) entitled "Queen for a Day?" Avoid settling for a day. Rather, choose to be king or queen for a lifetime—yours!

Pursue high-level-healthiness. Learn to love yourself for who you are. Take control of your life. If you need help, work with a healthcare professional or life coach. Choose to be happy. Find ways to do what you love. Give back and leave this planet better than you found it.

The twelfth key factor is sleep. Turn to the next chapter and discover how sleep is independently linked with longevity.

Be Brain Wise

It's a myth that you can cheat successfully on the amount of sleep you get. You may train yourself to 'get by' on less, but your brain will pay the price in the long term.

Sleep is independently linked with longevity. Early to bed and early to rise can help you stay healthier, make wiser choices, slow the onset of symptoms of aging, and potentially extend your years—to say nothing of keeping life in those years.

Key Factor—12
Sustaining Shuteye

The reward of sleep is often recognized by its absence.

—Robert Ornstein PhD and David Sobel MD

"Sleep. What's that?" asked Marilyn, grimacing humorously. "I'm lucky if I get 4 or 5 hours a night. There is just so much that *must* be done!"

"I suggest you re-evaluate what *must* be done," her physician replied. "Early to bed and early to rise is not an 'old wives' tale. Losing sleep is negatively impacting your brain-body health, your weight, and your longevity. Dr. James B. Maas pointed out in his book *Power Sleep,* that healthy sleep has been proven to be the single most important determinant in predicting longevity. If you want to be around to play with your grandchildren and maybe even your great grandchildren, something in your life must change and change quickly." Marilyn slumped dejectedly in her chair. "Let me hit a few highpoints about sleep. Listen carefully." The doctor summarized.

The loss of one hour per night of sleep over many nights has subtle cognitive costs that appear to go unrecognized by the sleep-deprived individual, while more severe loss of sleep for a week leads to profound cognitive deficits similar to those seen in some stroke patients—which also appear to go unrecognized by the individual. —University of Kansas

Loss of sleep results in chemical changes that deplete the immune system, increase growth of fat rather than muscle, accelerate the aging process and memory impairment, increase the risk for depression, and are linked with bone and cardiovascular tissue damage. —Eve Van Cauter

The brain's pre-frontal cortex contains complex executive functions related to emotional control, decision making, and social behavior. Sleep deprivation may lead to aggressive or bullying behaviors, delinquency, or even substance abuse.
—University of Michigan Medical School

A side-sleeping position seems to improve clearance of wastes from the brain. —Stony Brook University

The brain's prefrontal cortex is always active when you are awake and regenerates itself during sleep. It is very sensitive to sleep deprivation—which can impair its ability to regulate emotional expression that is necessary to control irritability, anger, and aggression. Sleep deprived individuals are more easily irritated, more likely to be angry, more likely to blame others, and are even more likely to plan revenge.
—American Academy of Sleep Medicine

Sleep requirements tend to remain constant throughout adulthood. New evidence shows that sleep is essential to mood, memory, cognitive performance, creativity, immune function, weight management, and longevity. Each brain has an optimum amount of sleep that it needs on a daily basis. Infants generally require about 16 hours, teenagers 9, and most adults 7 to 8 hours. —National Sleep Foundation

"I had no idea," said Marilyn. "Changes are starting tonight."

Sleep Cycle

The human wake-sleep cycle consists of roughly 8 hours of nocturnal sleep and 16 hours of daytime wakefulness. A complete sleep cycle consists of several sleep stages, each of which consists of a combination of both Rapid Eye Movement (REM) and non-REM sleep. Your sleep cycle is controlled by a combination of two internal influences: sleep homeostasis (the process by which the body maintains a steady state of internal conditions); and circadian rhythms (cyclical changes that occur over 24 hours and are driven by the brain's internal biological clock).

Different parts of the brain rest during different stages of the sleep cycle—sleep cannot be cut short without potentially interfering with critical brain functions. Loss of even a few hours of sleep during the night, can interfere with needed repairs to neurons, lower the production of neurotrophins (neuron food), and prompt the immune system to turn against healthy tissue and organs.

The human brain responds to its environment and appears to function best in sync with the circadian rhythm. There is something to be said for going to bed with the dark and waking up with the light. When people impose a variation of this circadian rhythm on the brain by going to bed too late, real health consequences can occur, including increased risks for increased anxiety and autoimmune diseases.

Gender Differences

Nan Hee Kim MD PhD studied sleep-deprived males and females and identified some disturbing results.

Sleep-deprived males were more likely to have diabetes or sarcopenia (an age-related loss of muscle strength and mobility), compared with males who obtained sufficient amounts of sleep. Females with sleep deficits tended to have more belly fat and an increased risk of metabolic syndrome, which raised their risk of heart disease, stroke, and diabetes. Independent of lifestyle, those who went to bed later at night had a higher risk of developing health problems as compared with those who were 'early-to-bed and early-to-rise'—even when both groups got the same amount of sleep overall.

Sleep-Obesity Link

Stress from sleep-deprivation can trigger the stress response. High levels of the stress hormone, cortisol, are linked with cravings for fatty snacks. Columbia University researchers found that those with insufficient sleep tended to eat an extra 300 calories a day. Both genders ate more protein-rich foods but only females ate more fat—an average of 31 more grams of fat after sleeping only four hours. According to University of Chicago researchers, the marked decrease in average sleep duration over the last 50 years coincides with the increase in prevalence of obesity worldwide—a pandemic.

The Wisconsin Sleep Cohort Study found that too little sleep altered levels of appetite-regulating hormones. When tired from lack of sleep, doing energy-intensive tasks, or dealing with high-maintenance people, many may further stress their brain by snacking on high fat, high sugar, fast food items, or beverages with high levels of sugar and caffeine or alcohol. These types of responses do little to alleviate brain fatigue but can do a great deal to increase one's weight.

Sleep Sick

Stanford professor Dr. William C. Dement, author of *The Promise of Sleep,* identified sleep deprivation as the most common brain impairment and says "We are a sleep-sick society." He regularly challenges his students to identify the optimum amount of sleep for their brains and to adopt a sleep-smart lifestyle. Guesstimate how much sleep you think your brain needs (e.g., seven or eight hours). Then get more sleep than that for several nights in a row. Eventually, your brain will begin to wake up spontaneously when it has had sufficient sleep. Make a note of the number of hours, which typically represent your brain's optimum sleep needs. Then give your brain the quantity and quality of sleep it needs on a daily basis. Otherwise, you can accumulate a sleep debt that can be difficult if not impossible to pay back.

Fewer than seven hours of sleep at night has been associated with a decrease in overall blood flow to the brain. Studies have shown a growing link between sleep duration and a variety of serious health problems, including diabetes, hypertension, depression, and obesity.

Sleep-Deprived Intoxication

After 20 hours without sleep your brain functions as it does at the legal blood alcohol limit in the State of California (.08). Fatigue is believed to have contributed to both the Exxon Valdez and space shuttle Challenger disasters. Motorist sleepiness accounts for 33 percent of traffic accidents. In some countries, sleep deprivation accounts for an estimated $16 billion in annual medical costs.

David K. Randall points out in *Dreamland*, that within the first 24 hours of sleep deprivation, the person's blood pressure begins to rise, then metabolism processes start to go haywire, resulting in an uncontrollable craving for carbohydrates. Soon the body temperature drops and the immune system gets weaker. If this goes on for too long, there is a good chance that the mind will turn against itself, triggering brain phenomenon in which the person experiences visions and hears phantom sounds akin to a bad acid trip.

Mental skills suffer severely from sleep deprivation, even more so than physical skills. The ability to make simple decisions or recall obvious facts drops off severely—even though the sleep-deprived individual does not seem to recognize the decrease in mental ability. Concentration is only 70 percent of what it is on days when the brain is well-rested. It is a bizarre downward spiral that is all the more peculiar because it can be stopped (if it isn't too late) by sleeping.

Sleep Tips

Arthur Schopenhauer offers an interesting perspective. He says that sleep is the interest we have to pay on the capital which is called in at death; and the higher the rate of interest and the more regularly it is paid, the further the date of redemption is postponed.

The National Sleep Foundation offers tips for getting the optimum amount of restful sleep your brain needs on a regular basis. Here are a few suggestions, some of which can be found on their website.

- Train yourself to associate certain restful activities with sleep (e.g., warm bath or shower, reading time) and make them part of your bedtime ritual. Turn off all electronics at least one hour before going to bed.

- Go to bed at the same time each night and get up at the same time each morning. Maximize the benefits of sleep by keeping your weekday and weekend sleeping schedule and routines similar.

- Develop techniques such as contemplative relaxation to quiet a 'racing mind.' Practice them at bedtime or after awakening during the night.

- If you lost an hour of sleep the night before, try to get a 15-minute power nap the next afternoon.

Sleep is absolutely necessary for survival. Far from being unproductive time, sleep plays a direct role in how full, energetic, and successful your life can be. What you think you achieve by reducing sleep is likely an illusion both in the amount and quality of work performed.

The number one recommendation from the California Human Population Laboratory Study for living longer and in better health—was sleep. Obtaining sufficient sleep is a key principle over which you can have a great deal of control. Stop rationalizing and kidding yourself. Adopt a sleep-smart lifestyle—now. As the old saying goes, the life you save may be your own.

The thirteenth key factor addresses the power of play and relaxation. Turn to the next chapter.

Be Brain Wise

Consciously build opportunities into your schedule on a regular basis for relaxation, play, and laughter. Not only can these healthy pleasures add fun and relaxation to your life, they can also assist in age-proofing your brain.

Think of these healthy pleasures as 'power plays.' Consistently give them to your brain. It will love them—and you for providing them!

Key Factor—13
Power Plays

Relaxation means releasing all concern and tension and letting the natural order of life flow through one's being.

—Donald Curtis

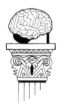 "Betsy!" exclaimed Linnie, seeing her friend in the check-out line at the supermarket. "I picked up the most amazing paperback at the school's book sale last week. You absolutely must read it."

"What's the title?" asked Betsy.

"*Healthy Pleasures,*" said Linnie. "Do you remember that old proverb about all work and no play?"

"Sure do," said Betsy. "Let's see what I can recall:

All work and no play makes you a dull boy.
All play and no work makes you a mere toy.

"I remember being upset that it talked only about a 'boy.'" Betsy laughed. "So I wrote my own version. It wasn't a great verse but at least it was about a girl! Let me think . . . see if I can remember how it went."

All work and no play, I'm a dismal girl.
All play and no work, I'm an unfinished pearl.

"That's cute," said Linnie. "How old were you?"

"Oh, seven or eight," said Betsy. "I lived with my elderly grandparents, you know. I know they loved me and did their best to take good care of me but their perspective was that 'idle hands are the devil's workshop.' As a child, work was always emphasized. Never play. I don't even remember getting to play. As an adult, I definitely know how to work. On the other hand, I'm quite sure I don't really know how to play and tend to feel guilty whenever I even try."

"I heard a documentary not long ago that said the brain loves to play. The brain-function specialist called fun and relaxation activities 'power plays.' And while 'play is the work of children,' the adult brain need play and relaxation, too. Did you know that scientists like Einstein would work for a while and then do something different for relaxation? And while they were 'playing,' their brain was still thinking about their 'work' subconsciously and would often come up with solutions and great ideas after a 'power-play' break."

"What else did *Healthy Pleasures* say?" asked Betsy.

"I'll lend it to you today," said Linnie. "It's very clear that all work and no play makes for deadly dull and dreary. To say nothing of: dark, dingy, disconsolate, dismal, drab, depressing, dreary, and you name it."

"How do you do that?" asked Betsy. "How in the wide-wide world do you come up with a string of words like that, just off the top of your head, so to speak?"

"It's just my brain *playing*," said Linnie, "and it is great fun."

"Read the book, Betsy" Linnie continued, "and then we can talk about it together. It's really important to include healthy pleasures in your routine every day."

"I'll read it right away," said Betsy. "I do need to get more balance in my life. I know that. My doctor was all over my case last week and told me to 'Lighten up and put some fun in your life, for heaven's sake!' Apparently it's one way to manage stress effectively. I'm ready to learn."

Many studies have confirmed that giving your brain time to relax from life's hectic pace can be of great benefit. Much like the rest of your body, your brain will eventually succumb to aging. However, you can do something to slow down the process. There are many people in their 80s and 90s and older who still have sharp memories and acute cognitive skills. Studies suggest that engaging in healthy pleasures on a regular basis can help retard the onset of symptoms of aging.

Many people find great satisfaction in their work. Relaxation involves a different type of satisfaction. The purpose of relaxation activities is to reduce tension. Therefore, it is important to utilize relaxation strategies that work with your brain and your pleasure. Yes, your pleasure.

In their book *Healthy Pleasures,* authors Robert Ornstein PhD and David Sobel MD, write about a new approach to managing your health. The bottom line is how important it is to include activities in your life that give you healthy pleasure and to expect pleasure from them. This includes relaxation.

You don't have time for relaxation activities? Think again! According to author Sydney J. Harris, the time to relax is when you don't have time for it.

Relax instead of worrying. Take a lesson from Mark Twain who reportedly said, "I've had a lot of troubles in my life, most of which never happened." Worry and anxiety are forms of fear and never help with problem solving or sound sleep or rewarding relationships or health, or a host of other undesirable behaviors and outcomes.

Leonardo da Vinci believed in relaxation and recommended it. He wrote:

> *Every now and then go away, have a little relaxation, for when you come back to your work your judgment will be surer. Go some distance away because then the work appears smaller and more of it can be taken in at a glance and a lack of harmony and proportion is more readily seen.*

Pay attention to what your brain enjoys. Identify the healthy pleasures that are tension and stress releasers for your brain. Give yourself those gifts on a regular basis. On a regular *daily* basis.

Relax Creatively

Be creative. Every brain is creative—even ones that have been told they're not. An old Chinese proverb goes like this:

> *Tension is who you think you should be—relaxation is who you are.*

No doubt there are as many ways to relax as there are individual brains living on this planet. Find the strategies that work well for your brain. Here are a few ideas to get you started. Remember, the sky is the limit!

- Take a break and do some alternate activity. Take a mini-vacation for a few hours or for a day. A change can be as good as a rest.

- Listen to music or play music if you have a favorite musical instrument. Sing or exercise your vocal chords in a karaoke bar. Identify the type of music that relaxes and thrills your brain. The release of endorphins from engaging in some form of music can actually induce a state of musical euphoria.

- Close your eyes and clear your mind of stressors. Concentrate on brain breathing for a few minutes.

- Do what you enjoy, such as playing board games with your family, enrolling in a painting class, having lunch with a dear friend or some other preferred activity.

- Sniff some spiced-apple fragrance—a scent that has been associated with a relaxed but alert brain state.

- If you enjoy writing, keep a 'journal' in hardcopy or electronic. Write prose or poetry. Compose a song. Jot down reminiscences from childhood or wishes to put in your bucket list.

- Devote an hour to your favorite hobby. Don't have one? Get one!

Choose to Be Happy

Is your brain happy? According to St. Thomas Aquinas, '*It is requisite for the relaxation of the mind that we make use, from time to time, of playful deeds and jokes.*'

Happiness likely correlates with how much time a person spends feeling good rather than with specific events. Hang out with happy people. Choose to be happy. It's relaxing! Think of something about which to be grateful. It's physiologically impossible to be grateful and fearful at the same time.

Have fun. Laugh often. If you can laugh at yourself, you'll have an unending supply of triggers. Mirthful laughter is good medicine and can be healing to both brain and body. It can alter your neurochemistry positively, increasing your levels of serotonin, dopamine, and endorphins. It can help your food digest better. It even releases substances that help with constipation. Who knew?

Relaxation Techniques

If you simply cannot relax, you may be one who could benefit from specific relaxation techniques. These strategies can include deep muscle relaxation or massage, meditation, guided imagery, or biofeedback. Studies on a variety of relaxation strategies have shown physiological changes as people relax. Some of these observed changes include a decreased heart rate, lower oxygen consumption, and slower sympathetic nervous system activity, such as is involved in the fight-flight response, for example.

Relaxation Response

The Relaxation Response (RR) is a strategy developed by Herbert Benson MD, Harvard Medical School professor and internationally known cardiologist. The benefits that can be derived from this contemplative exercise—and there are many—are documented in his best-selling book *The Relaxation Response.*

Briefly, four basic elements underlay the elicitation of the Relaxation Response, regardless of the cultural source. These four elements are:

1. A quiet room or a relaxing outdoor location

2. A thought or object upon which to concentrate

3. A choice of attitude (e.g., eliminate distractions and other thoughts from your mind, avoid mind-wandering)

4. A comfortable position (e.g., sitting)

Practice the Relaxation Response for ten to twenty minutes each day and watch your life improve. You are the only person that can choose relaxation and play—healthy pleasures—for your brain. Even a short walk in nature can be relaxing and play for your brain. Imagine how your brain will enjoy a break, thrill to be doing something different, appreciate an activity it loves doing, and be grateful that you care enough about it to take good care of it.

What about aerobic exercises for the brain? Key factor number fourteen addresses those. They are waiting for you.

Be Brain Wise

Be proactive. Obtain at least thirty minutes of challenging mental exercise on a daily basis. Read aloud for at least ten minutes every day. Reading aloud is much more stimulating for your brain than reading silently and is an inexpensive way to exercise your brain.

Remember, the brain loves novelty and is stimulated by variety and whatever is new. Be sure to hang out with smart people.

Key Factor—14
Brain Exercise

*As with muscles, you can strengthen your neural pathways
with brain exercise or you can let them wither. The
principle is the same: use it or lose it!*

—John J. Ratey MD

"My brain seems to be slowing down," Anita
said. "That's downright scary! My neighbor just
bought a computer and is taking some classes on
line. 'To exercise my brain,' as she put it."

"I attended a seminar recently and learned that
challenging mental stimulation—brain aerobic exercise they
called it—is an anti-aging strategy," her friend Rosie replied.
"Studies in several different countries have shown that more
education appears to lower your risk for some dementias."

"My family managed to send my older brother to college,
but not me or my three sisters," said Anita. "Then I got
married and children came along and we were all so busy …
I wonder if it would do any good now. I've always wanted
to write, you know, an article or a story or even a book. But
I'm probably too old to consider going back to school."

"Of course you're not too old—unless you tell yourself you
are. The speaker said it's never too late to do something to
challenge and stimulate your brain," said Rosie.

"As long as you still have a functioning brain," Rosie added, laughing. "Do what your neighbor is doing. I know there are writing classes on line."

"We do have a computer," said Anita. "But so far all I've done is stand there and look at it." She laughed, ruefully.

"I heard that learning how to use a computer and doing an Internet search can be as challenging for an older brain as reading a book. That's a wow!" said Rosie. "We've talked about getting one. I think this will tip us over the edge and get it done. It's not about a diploma or a degree unless that's one of your goals. It is about ongoing challenging mental stimulation and learning that can help age-proof your brain."

Stimulate Your Brain

Mental stimulation is definitely one of the factors over which you have some control. Sarah Yang reported that researchers at UC Berkeley found a significant association between higher levels of cognitive (mental) activity over a lifetime and lower levels of beta-amyloid, that destructive protein that is the hallmark of Alzheimer's disease. While previous research suggested that engaging in mentally stimulating activities (e.g., reading, writing, and playing games) may help stave off Alzheimer's later in life, the UC Berkley study showed how stimulating brain activities seem to decrease the levels of beta-amyloid.

Positron Emission Tomography (PET Scans) revealed that people with no symptoms of Alzheimer's, who had engaged in cognitively stimulating activities throughout their lives, had fewer deposits of beta-amyloid.

Multiple studies have shown that brain activity helps new connections form in the brain. It turns out that brain activity is needed for selecting which synapses should be eliminated, as well. The findings have implications for conditions in which these mechanisms may have gone awry (e.g., autism, schizophrenia, and perhaps Alzheimer's).

Almost daily another piece of research confirms how critically important it is for you to keep your brain challenged, stimulated, and active! Roni Caryn Rabin pointed out in her article, *"For a Sharp Brain, Stimulation,"* that there is consensus among scientists on a few recommendations for action to help preserve brain function. These include physical activity, Mediterranean-style cuisine, avoiding head injuries, staying away from pesticides, trying new things, and cognitive or mental training.

Studies in the United Kingdom led by Bob Woods found consistent evidence from multiple trials that cognitive stimulation programs, 45 minutes 5 times a week for a total of 225 minutes, benefited cognition in people with mild to moderate dementia over and above any medication effects. Others are suggesting 30 minutes of challenging mental exercise a day as a possible prevention strategy.

Scientists agree that preventing brain deficits will always be easier than restoring them. The sooner you get on board with age-proofing your brain, the more there may be to save. The sooner you can intervene, if that becomes necessary, the more likely you are to be successful. Embracing a program to improve memory and slow down symptoms of brain aging requires avoiding denial and accepting that you need such a program. Everyone does.

Neurons

Your brain is unique, is capable of making an unlimited number of synaptic connections, can learn seven facts per second, every second, for the rest of your life and still have plenty of room left over to learn more—and will improve with age if you use it properly. —Michael Gelb

Although not muscles, neurons respond much like muscle tissue; they tend to atrophy with disuse and become stronger with exercise. *Use it or lose it* is the mantra for brain-function in the 21st Century! Look at the neuron drawings below: each has a cell body, a long axon projecting from the cell body, and many small finger-like projections known as dendrites—which help pull information into the neurons so you can 'think' about it.

One neuron has received regular stimulation and one has not. How do you want your neurons to look?

It is believed possible to grow

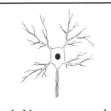

1. Neuron exposed to low levels of mental stimulation

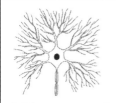

2. Neuron exposed to high levels of mental stimulation

10,000 dendrites on one neuron. The more dendrites on a neuron the more connections it can make with other neurons. Learning new information or doing something in a new way can give your dendrites a workout. You can alter the shape of a dendrite in thirty (30) seconds and grow a new one in thirty (30) minutes depending on what you are doing and how challenging and stimulating the activity is to your brain.

Brain research has provided conclusions that serve as a basis for anti-aging brain strategies, especially in terms of effective brain exercises. What you do or don't do to stimulate your neurons can make a difference! Without regular stimulation through challenging mental exercise, axons and dendrites can shrink, widening the space (synapse) between neurons. This can accelerate the aging process and lead to symptoms of senility or dementia. The more active your neurons, the more neurotrophins or brain food the supporting glial cells produce and the more responsive the neurons are to it.

Solving 'Brain Benders' is touted as a whole-brain exercise. So is travel, local or abroad. Being exposed to new places, music, sounds, foods, odors, languages, architecture, vehicles, clothing, furniture, temperatures, topography, flora and fauna, and customs all stimulate your brain. You can also stimulate your brain by altering your routines and trying something in a new way. Use your opposite hand when doing tasks such as brushing your teeth, combing your hair, eating with your fork, stirring your hot drink, or using your phone or remote. Turn all the pictures on your desk or bureau upside down for a few days. Pay attention to what your brain does with that! You may be really surprised.

Stimulate your brain with music and make it a regular part of your brain's life. Do you play a musical instrument? Do so for a few minutes every day. Do you like to sing? Join a choir. Or compose, arrange, hum, and whistle; attend musical programs, plays, and symphonies. The sky is the limit unless you limit yourself. And typically you are limited only by your reticence to try something new or do something in a new way.

Challenging Mental Exercise

Stimulate your left cerebral hemisphere through:

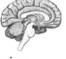

- Crossword and scrambled-words puzzles
- Smiling and laughing a lot every day
- Reading and listening to audiobooks
- Memorizing poems and/or prose that you enjoy
- Find-the-word puzzles and/or simple math problems

Stimulate your right cerebral hemisphere through:

- Map reading and mazes
- Jigsaw and 3D puzzles
- Games that match colors and objects
- Jokes and other humorous activities
- Travel, locally or abroad

Whole-brain strategies include:

- Figuring out 'Brain Benders' (www.arlenetaylor.org)
- Solving riddles and doing 'Daffynitions'
- Working Sudoku-type puzzles
- Telling a joke and choosing to laugh about it

There are any number of apps available with games that can stimulate and challenge your brain. The joy of solving brain puzzles often comes from pushing yourself to make a mental leap (away from existing assumptions) and to explore other possibilities you might once have thought impossible. When a specific mental exercise is no longer challenging, move up to the next level, or find a different and more challenging activity, and so on.

Your Mental Exercise Program

The possibilities for challenging mental exercise are virtually endless. Just be sure to get variety, including things that are new and different. Here are some ideas.

- Count to a hundred as fast as you can, then count backwards. Do simple math problems, then try to beat your own time.

- Write poems, stories, limericks, songs, books, articles, or you name it. Memorize new verses and prose passages.

- Develop a new hobby or learn a foreign language. Travel to your destination by an alternate route—on purpose.

- Do the mental exercises in the book *Age-Proofing Your Memory* or something similar. Look for brain-aerobic exercises. They're out there.

- Join a reading club. Increasing your reading speed can help your brain become more active. Read aloud for ten minutes a day. Reading aloud stimulates more of your brain than reading silently, and you also exercise your tongue, teeth, mouth, and larynx or voice box.

It's your brain and it is up to you to exercise it. No one can do this for you and it can make the difference between a vibrant healthy longevity or (you fill in the blank).

The fifteenth key factor is next: ***Potent 20:80 Rule.*** Don't know what that is? Turn the page and find out.

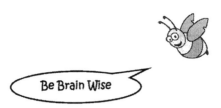

Be Brain Wise

Develop, implement, and hone effective stress-managements strategies. Include strategies such as Brain Breathing and the Quieting Reflex as stress reducers. In combination, these strategies can be powerful.

Live the 20:80 Rule on a consistent basis. You'll be glad you did—because it can make a positive difference in your life.

Key Factor—15
Potent 20:80 Rule

Adopting the right attitude can convert a negative stress into a positive one.

—Dr. Hans Selye

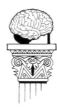 "Stress, stress, and more stress!" exclaimed Aretha. "Planning this wedding for our daughter is so stressful! I don't know if I'm coming or going. At night I lay awake ruminating about this and that and the other thing and what could go wrong…"

"It's just a wedding, for heaven's sake," said her husband, Dave. "Chill. Relax. Take a deep breath. Get over it."

"Ah-h-h, you may need more than a deep breath," said his brother Tom, visiting from overseas. "Unmanaged stress is lethal to both brain and body. Did you know it can actually kill brain cells?" Aretha and Dave shook their heads. "Effective stress-management strategies are important for everyone but especially for females because their brains are twice as vulnerable as male brains to many stress-related disorders including depression and PTSD (posttraumatic stress disorder). The female brain actually responds very differently to stressors when compared with the male brain."

"Hey Bro, are you saying that this wedding is more stressful for Aretha's brain than it is for mine?" asked Dave.

"The likelihood is yes, although stress is a relative concept and quite subjective," Tom replied. "You've heard the old saying: 'one person's pleasure is another's poison.' Recent rat-brain studies have shown that neurons in the locus ceruleus, an alarm center deep in the brainstem respond differently to Corticotropin Releasing Factor (CRF) in the female brain compared to the male brain. This powerful substance, both a hormone and a neurotransmitter, is released when a brain perceives a stressor."

"I knew it!" cried Aretha. "Here I'm hanging from the ceiling by my fingernails and Dave tells me to *chill. Relax. Get over it. Take a deep breath.*" She was not amused.

"It appears that the female brain has more difficulty coping with high levels of this CRF, which is both a hormone and a neurotransmitter," said Tom. "Our male brains have a unique adaptive process that prevents them from over-reacting so strongly to CRF, a strategy that does not occur in the female brain. For any given stressor, your brain, Dave, will likely under-react while Aretha's brain will likely over-react. In fact, researcher Debra Bangasser PhD has been reported as saying: 'Even in the absence of any stress, the female stress signaling system is more sensitive from the start.'"

"Well, who knew," said Dave. "What can I do to help?"

"Ask your wife," said Tom. "Ask her what her biggest stressor is right now and then listen carefully. Together you can craft a solution somewhere in the middle of your two perceptions. It's really worth the work." Dave looked at Aretha. She shrugged, still not amused.

"How about we meet for lunch tomorrow and do what Tom suggested?" Dave asked his wife.

Aretha started to say, "I don't have ..." but to her credit, she caught herself and replied instead, "Thanks for understanding, Dave. I'd like that."

Stress

Stress is part and parcel of living. A necessary phenomenon, it exists at all levels of life because simply being alive requires the brain and body to continually adapt to your external and internal worlds. Whenever anything changes in your life, your brain and body must respond. When they can no longer respond, you're history.

Definitions for *stress* abound and have evolved over time. One of the most commonly accepted definitions now—based on the work of Richard S. Lazarus PhD—is that stress is a condition, sense, or feeling that is experienced by individuals who perceive that the demands upon them exceed the personal and social resources they are able to mobilize. Stressors can be placed in one of three groups:

- Eustress – positive stress that can be healthy and valuable and can motivate you to grow and learn

- Distress – outright negative and undesirable stress that needs to be avoided or minimized whenever possible

- Misstress – stress that tends to be hidden so that its impact is often missed (e.g., too much sitting, long commutes, losing your keys repeatedly)

Unmanaged, distress and misstress can be killers. In fact, cumulatively, misstress can produce negative results that equal those of distress. In a state of distress there is no true relaxation between one stressful episode and the next. The stress response can become stuck in the '*on*' position, so to speak, a scenario often linked with mental, emotional, and physical ailments. Think of chronic stressors as the *trash* of modern life. Everyone generates some. Learn to *dispose* of it properly so it doesn't pile up and damage your life.

Stress and the Brain

If your teeth and fists are clenched and the muscles in your neck and back are tight and ropey, your brain probably is, too. That's because the brain is usually the first body system to recognize a stressor, reacting with split-second timing to instruct the body how to adjust. It can stimulate the stress response for as long as 72 hours after a traumatic incident. Longer if you continue to rehearse all the gory details. The bad news: unmanaged stress can cause brain damage. The good news: implementing effective stress-reduction strategies can enhance brain function.

Epictetus, a 2nd Century Greek philosopher, reportedly taught that it's not so much what happens to you that matters but what you think about what happens and the importance you place upon it. More recently, his perspective has been labeled the 20:80 Rule. In a nutshell, stressors are thought to interact with the brain in a two-part equation. Only 20 percent of the negative effect to the brain from a given situation is due to the event itself; 80 percent is due to your perception of the event and the importance or weight you give to it. What a powerful, practical, and potent concept!

You may not be able to do anything about the 20 percent—a specific event or situation. You can do almost everything about the 80 percent—your thoughts and the stories you tell yourself about that event or situation, the actions you take and the behaviors you exhibit. That's because your brain creates your own perceptions. To change the way you feel, you need to change the way you think.

Of course you need to be serious about life. But it is important not to take every little thing too seriously. That's where honing your sense of humor, including the ability to laugh at yourself and at the vagaries of life, can be so important. Laughter can decrease levels of cortisol released during episodes of stress. Just changing the muscles of your face into a smile promotes the release of feel-good brain chemicals such as endorphins. After all, the word 'stressed' is the word 'desserts' spelled backwards.

Break the Stress Cycle Quickly

Strategies to interrupt the stress cycle can include exercise, brain breathing, meditation, massage, a change of activities, and humor, to name just a few. They can also include the 6-second *Quieting Reflex* developed by Charles F. Stroebel MD, author of *QR, The Quieting Reflex.*

Designed to break the stress cycle, the *Quieting Reflex* can even be used to break patterns involving everyday stressful thoughts. Use the QR at the first sign of stress or tension, any time or any place. Practice until it becomes second-nature. There are just five simple steps.

1. Smile to counter facial tension and alter the brain's neurochemistry

2. Tell your brain and body you are alert and calm, even amused (use your given name and the pronoun you)

3. Breathe deeply and easily to increase the level of oxygen at the cellular level

4. Exhale and allow your body muscles to go limp as you feel warmth flowing through your body to your toes

5. Resume your normal activity

Bad News and Good News

In his book *The Brain That Changes Itself* Dr. Norman Doidge points out that 'essential cortical real estate' can be lost in response to illness, high stress, depression, and trauma. If the stress is brief, this decrease in size is temporary. If it is too prolonged, the damage is permanent. Scary thought—that the stress reaction creates specific hormonal imbalances that can damage or even kill brain cells, shrink brain tissue, and lead to symptoms of dementia and Alzheimer's disease. Other undesirable outcomes may include decreased ability to brainstorm options, altered brain neurochemistry, diminished self-esteem levels, negative mindset and self-talk, and emotional distress and depression.

Researchers have discovered that intentionally invoking positive emotions is one of the fastest and most effective ways to reduce unhealthy stress. Take gratitude and appreciation, components of the emotion of joy.

Dr. Rollin McCraty, Director of Research at the Institute of HeartMath, found that appreciation and gratitude are powerful stress-reducers. Heart-monitoring technology that measures heart-rhythm patterns typically displays a nearly instant transformation from erratic to smooth heart patterns when a person intentionally experiences appreciation. Smooth heart-rhythm patterns indicate lower stress and greater heart coherence, which provides a range of psychophysiological benefits that include improved memory, focus, and immune system function, among many others.

Become more aware in every moment of your life with an attitude of friendliness and compassion. Intentionally pay attention to what is happening around and within you. You are more likely to manage stress effectively when you understand how your brain and body function and when you identify how you learned to recognize, respond to, and manage stressors effectively. If you learned unhelpful stress-management strategies, learn new ones.

Identify *your* typical stressors and place them in one of the three main stressor categories: Eustress, Distress, and Misstress. Identify and dump as much distress and misstress as possible or minimize your exposure to them. Develop and consistently implement good stress-management strategies for the stressors you cannot avoid.

Now for key factor number sixteen: ***Emotional Intelligence Quotient*** or EQ for short. You may want to pay close attention to J-O-T behaviors.

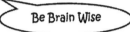

Be Brain Wise

Your level of EQ or Emotional Intelligence Quotient has a great deal to do with your success in life. Estimates are that EQ can contribute as much as eighty percent. It impacts all areas: mental, physical, emotional, spiritual, personal, professional, and social.

Dump J-O-T behaviors. Evaluate your own level of EQ. Raise it by honing your skills as needed to achieve positive outcomes on a more consistent basis—by design.

Key Factor—16
Emotional Intelligence Quotient

Emotional intelligence is not the opposite of intelligence, it is not the triumph of heart over head—it is the unique intersection of both.

—David Caruso

"Read my lips! I shall never, repeat *never*, speak to *that person* again. She was rude. Walked right past me in the store today without saying a word. I'm worth more than that, I tell you!" Carolyn was beyond indignant and on a roll. "I know one thing for sure and certain: I will not invite her to my party next month. She can find out what it feels like to be ignored. Dismissed out of hand. Let's see how she likes that?"

"That's a bit harsh, isn't it?" asked her neighbor. "I'd be willing to bet she never even noticed you today. Certainly she would have no reason to single you out to be ignored. After all I've never found her to be knowingly rude. Give it some time. Something may have happened to consume her attention." Sure enough, her neighbor was right.

Several weeks later the news leaked out that on the morning in question, *that person* had just found out her test results showed uterine cancer. At that, Carolyn did an about face. However, her brain and body had been negatively impacted by her weeks of bitterness and anger.

EQ and JOT

JOT is an acronym for three top symptoms often exhibited by individuals with low levels of emotional intelligence.

- J—stands for jumping to conclusions
- O—indicates overreacting to the event or situation
- T—means taking things personally

Would you like to live more successfully? Emotional Intelligence attempts to help people bring intelligence to emotion. EQ can be indispensable in handling relationships, enhancing creativity, and solving problems. Your success quotient or SQ is a combination of your IQ plus your level of EQ. But IQ and EQ don't contribute equally. Estimates are that IQ contributes a mere twenty percent to your success in life, while EQ contributes a solid eighty percent.

Top performers tend to use both in harmony. For example, successful managers tend to have high levels of EQ; less successful managers often have a high IQ but a low EQ.

Back to Carolyn. All things being equal, had she possessed a higher level of EQ she likely could have avoided the bitterness and anger she carried around for weeks, which spilled out all over everyone with whom she dealt. She likely would not have dismissed her friend out of hand, either. Unfortunately, Carolyn exhibited JOT behaviors big time. Equally unfortunate was the damage done to her own brain and body because of her reaction to the incident, to say nothing of a missed opportunity to provide emotional support to her friend (*that woman*)—had she sought her out and asked if everything was going okay for her.

EQ versus IQ

Dr. Daniel Goleman, in his book *Working with Emotional Intelligence*, defines EQ as the capacity for recognizing our own feelings and those of others, for motivating ourselves, and for managing emotions effectively in ourselves and in our relationships.

In their book *Handle with Care,* Anabel L. Jensen PhD and co-authors describe Emotional Intelligence as 'a way of recognizing, understanding, and choosing how we think, feel, and act.' That, instead of blindly exhibiting JOT behaviors.

In his book *Emotional Intelligence at Work*, Dahlip Singh PhD says that EQ consists of three psychological dimensions that motivate individuals to maximize productivity, manage change, and resolve conflict:

- Emotional sensitivity
- Emotional maturity
- Emotional competency

Learned Skills

The dimensions of a high EQ are skill-based as opposed to the inherited potential for IQ. EQ skills are learned and the good news is that they can be developed and honed at any stage of life. The earlier the better, of course, since estimates are that 50 percent of the problems most people face are of their own making, based on the way they think. Raise your EQ and watch many of your problems slip below the horizon of your life. Such a deal!

Unfortunately, the study of EQ has been largely ignored in educational institutions in favor of academic abilities. Also, unfortunately, society itself has failed to teach essential strategies for handling anger, resolving conflicts positively, maintaining impulse control, exhibiting empathy, and other key components of EQ.

You were very fortunate if your parents possessed and role-modeled high levels of EQ. That doesn't mean you chose to develop the skills but at least you were exposed to them and had the chance to experience how the skills worked. Many children don't have that opportunity because their parents and care providers and teachers didn't develop EQ skills—for whatever reason. You can only teach what you know.

Heart-EQ Connection

Studies have shown that the heart is more than just a collection of muscle cells as originally believed. It contains neurons, 40,000 or more. They look and function much as do brain neurons; use many of the same neurotransmitters; and eat similar neurotrophins (neuron food).

According to Doc Childre and Howard Martin, authors of *The HeartMath Solution,* and Dr. Paul Pearsall in *The Heart's Code,* what brain neurons are to IQ, heart neurons may be to EQ. A direct unmediated channel is believed to connect brain and heart neurons. Intelligence and intuition are thought to be heightened by input from heart neurons. Who knew? Because the heart is a subconscious organ, however, it often takes time for information to filter up from the heart to the brain and come to your conscious awareness.

Emotions versus Feelings

The words emotions and feelings are often used synonymously, but they actually represent different concepts and follow different pathways in the brain. Emotions usually surface automatically, based on some external or internal trigger. Feelings represent the brain's attempts to make sense of the emotions and interpret their import. This means that while you are not always responsible for every emotion that surfaces, you need to take responsibility for the feelings you maintain (because your brain created them) and for any actions you take based on your feelings.

Observable Behaviors

In addition to positive-mindset and self-talk patterns, self-awareness, and motivational abilities, individuals with high levels of EQ tend to exhibit some specific behavioral characteristics. Generally they are able to:

- Identify, label accurately, assess intensity, and express emotions appropriately

- Recognize what the emotion is signaling or trying to communicate

- Exhibit effective verbal and nonverbal skills, along with empathy and compassion

- Articulate the difference between recognizing and identifying a specific emotion and taking action based on that emotion

- Listen, read, and interpret social cues and understand the perspective of others whether or not there is agreement

- Delay gratification and exhibit good impulse control

- Manage their own feelings and moods effectively

- Handle relationships effectively, avoiding or minimizing any tendency to jump to conclusions, overreact, or take things personally

Help Your Brain

There can be a huge difference in behaviors between persons with low versus high levels of emotional intelligence. High EQ can impact your life in many positive ways. Potentially it can assist you in maintaining good cognitive brain function and enable you to avoid specific problems that could result in negative outcomes. Studies have shown that high levels of EQ may help you:

- Reduce or mitigate the effects of undesirable stressors
- Minimize conflict and enhance your relationships
- Improve your life personally and professionally
- Realize a sense of personal empowerment
- Role-model a more effective way to live

The bad news is that most educational systems do not teach EQ skills. You're somehow expected to pick them up on your own. The good news is that learning EQ skills is a choice. You can develop and/or raise your EQ at any time and at any age if you choose to do so.

Trauma Connection

Some researchers believe the brain can stop developing emotionally at the time it experiences a traumatic event, including physical or sexual abuse—especially when the trauma is reoccurring and the brain doesn't know how to recover or doesn't have the appropriate help to do so. Naturally, this may interfere with the brain's development of EQ skills. Consequently, some may have an emotional age that is lower than their chronological age, a situation that can contribute to a plethora of problems in both personal and professional arenas. With effective recovery strategies, as the brain heals from the trauma, it may again continue to develop emotionally and learn helpful EQ skills.

You can plot behaviors on a metaphorical continuum based on their relative positive or negative outcomes.

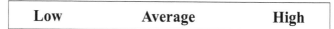

Low	Average	High

The higher your own level of EQ, usually the easier it is to recognize low versus high EQ behaviors—in yourself and in others. Compare your typical behaviors against characteristics that represent high levels of EQ. Have you been exhibiting any JOT behaviors lately? Evaluate your emotional age. You may need to raise your EQ so that it matches (or even exceeds) your chronological age. Start honing EQ skills now, live more effectively, and watch your life improve.

Time to move on to key factor number seventeen. Are you using natural light regularly and judiciously? Check out the next chapter.

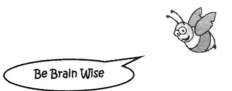

Be Brain Wise

Light up your life and your brain with natural light. Live in rooms that are sunny and bright or compensate with natural full-spectrum lighting.

On the other hand, protect your skin from sun damage. Be judicious about the amount of exposure you get to direct sunlight. Avoid tanning parlors. Use sunglasses regularly, a strategy that may help to prevent macular degeneration.

Key Factor—17
Lifesaving Light

Live in rooms full of light.

—Cornelius Celsus

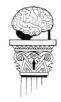 The shadows lengthened, creating interesting patterns on the forest floor. The lake rippled gently in the evening breeze. On the far side of the lake, Old Sol (a name for the sun in several languages) seemed to move ever faster toward the horizon. "This reminds me of my childhood," said Granny, wistfully. "My dad brought us to this lake the year I turned ten. For my birthday. It's lovely to be back here again with all of you."

"And now I'm ten," said precocious Rebekah, sighing happily, "and you brought me here." She looked at the family members gathered around the fire pit, waiting for the campfire to be lit and burst into flame at sunset. Calico, the little Border collie, sat beside Rebekah, its head on her knee, watching the light of life continue its inexorable journey downward toward the horizon.

"There are no clouds tonight," said Granny. "It's just possible we'll see a *green flash* as the sun slips below the level of the lake. Now that would be treat. Keep your eyes on the horizon, Rebekah. That great ball of liquid fire looks as if it's just ready to dip into the water. If it happens it'll only be for a few seconds." Rebekah held her breath.

Sure enough. As darkness fell from the wings of night, in the words of Granny's favorite poet, they were rewarded with a lovely green flash that lasted for just a few seconds before the sun slipped from sight. Almost immediately, Calico flopped down on the ground, gave a contented sigh much as Rebekah had done, and fell sound asleep.

"Calico goes to sleep when the sun sets," said Rebekah.

"It's her biological clock," said Rebekah's father.

"What's a biological clock?" asked Rebekah, interested. "Do I have one?"

"Certainly," her father replied. "All biologic beings do. Your 'clock' is located in your brain's hypothalamus in a tiny area about the size of a grain of rice that's shaped like a pine cone. Known as the suprachiasmatic nucleus or SCN for short; it contains about 20,000 neurons that respond automatically to the circadian rhythms of day and night, light and dark. Your clock regulates the routine changes in the functions of your brain and body that occur over the course of 24 hours. This includes sleep and wakefulness."

"My teacher says her watch runs on the light of the sun," said Rebekah, "but it doesn't fall asleep when it gets dark out."

"That's because it stores energy from the sun, which allows it to keep ticking away even when it's dark out," explained Granny. "My father had a pocket watch that had to be wound regularly. Then batteries were invented. Now there's a special system that works from sunlight." She shook her head. "Technologies certainly have come a long way."

Life Sustaining

Plants cannot survive without sunlight. Neither can you. For Greeks and Romans in the ancient world, Apollo was the god of sun and light and healing. Because of the rays of the sun, sighted creatures can *see* the world around them. Even seeing *by the light of the moon* involves Old Sol. Sunlight impacts your 24-hour biological clock and its rhythm encourages nighttime sleep. It also allows many people to awaken rested and with no help from either a rooster or an alarm clock.

When light enters your eye, it activates neurons in the retina that convert photons (light particles) to electrical signals. These signals travel along the optic nerve to the 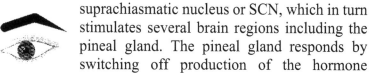 suprachiasmatic nucleus or SCN, which in turn stimulates several brain regions including the pineal gland. The pineal gland responds by switching off production of the hormone melatonin, and this makes you feel more awake. The SCN also governs your body temperature, hormone secretion, urine production, and changes in blood pressure. After darkness falls, the SCN signals once again and your body's level of melatonin increases, making you feel drowsy.

Sunlight is the most effective regulator of your brain's biological clock. Even going to bed after midnight has a nearly immediately effect of dysregulating your natural circadian rhythms covered by your suprachiasmatic nucleus or biological clock. The consequences of this may lead to insomnia, a harder time falling asleep, or difficulty staying asleep. Even if you have a schedule that permits you to sleep in, your quality of sleep may not be as good.

Anything that disrupts its light-sensitive circadian rhythms can have a far-reaching impact on your brain's and body's abilities to function effectively. This includes shift work. Studies have shown that night-shift workers, despite having a schedule that allows for an adequate amount of sleep, obtain less sleep than those who work days. It also includes problems related to jet lag due to travel as the brain is carried quickly into another time zone, when the times for sunset and sunrise may be hours different from where you live. And it includes adults with a sleep-disrupted infant who sleeps all day and cries all night, which naturally leads to sleep-disrupted parents and care providers.

Seasonal Affective Disorder (SAD)

Some people are so sensitive to light or the lack therefore that they experience seasonal changes in feelings of well-being based on the time of year and amount of available sunlight. They may do quite well for the couple of months every year, May 21st to July 21st for example, when the sun doesn't deign to sink below the horizon. Conversely, six months later when the sun changes its mind and barely rises above the horizon, the days are much shorter. Light-sensitive individuals can develop symptoms that can run the gamut from carbohydrate cravings and weight gains, to anxiety, diminished energy, decreased physical activity, an increased need for sleep, and depression.

Norman E. Rosenthal MD, internationally recognized for his work in depression research and author of *Winter Blues,* coined the term Seasonal Affective Disorder or SAD to describe the difficulties that some individuals experience when they are exposed to inadequate amounts of sunlight.

Dr. Rosenthal estimates that about six percent of Americans experience seasonal difficulties along with others living in parts of Norway, Finland, Alaska, and Iceland, to name just a few. The University of Anchorage studied residents of Fairbanks and discovered that 28 percent reported symptoms of SAD. Areas of Maine and Minnesota reported even higher rates—30 percent, while New York reported ten percent and Florida reported only two percent.

If you think you might be one of these light-sensitive individuals, be sure to consult a healthcare professional. Fortunately there are remedies for SAD such as 'natural or full-spectrum lighting' for both home and work environments. Studies have shown multiple benefits, including less perceptual fatigue and better visual acuity.

If you need more natural light than others or need to *light up* your life a bit brighter, here are some suggestions:

- Trim bushes around the windows to allow more natural light to enter.

- Paint walls and ceilings light colors or off-white to keep the interior of home bright. Hang mirrors to enhance the light.

- Purchase and use a commercial light box or use natural or full-spectrum lighting or install skylights.

- Exercise outdoors, when possible. When exercising indoors do so in the presence of natural or full-spectrum lighting.

Melatonin-Light Connection

Melatonin is a hormone secreted by the pineal gland in the brain. Its secretion follows a daily rhythm governed by your body's biological clock. When you are exposed to sunlight or very bright artificial light in the morning, your nocturnal melatonin production occurs sooner. Consequently, although melatonin doesn't control sleep per se, you may enter into sleep more easily at night. Healthy young and middle-aged adults usually secrete between five and twenty-five micrograms of melatonin each night. Night melatonin production may be impacted by the modern-day penchant for indoor activity and for staying up well past dusk. In addition, melatonin secretion tends to decline with age—a possible link with an observed age-related rise in difficulty sleeping for some elderly adults.

According to Russel J. Reiter PhD, melatonin researcher at the University of Texas Health Science Center and author of the book *Melatonin—Your Body's Natural Wonder Drug:*

> *The light we get from being outside on a summer day can be a thousand times brighter than we're ever likely to experience indoors.*

Benefits of Sunlight

Sunlight triggers an increase in serotonin, the feel-good brain chemical that controls sleep patterns and body temperature. It can also lift your mood, ward off depression, positively impact your sex drive, and increase levels of endorphins (natural morphine) in the brain.

Natural sunlight triggers the body to make its own vitamin D, which is crucial to health. Some estimate that ten to fifteen minutes of sun exposure a day is sufficient for most people to generate Vitamin D for that day. Too much exposure, on the other hand, can damage collagen and destroy Vitamin A in the skin and increase the risk of skin cancer due to changes in cellular DNA.

Studies in schools, classrooms, and other work environments where people spend time learning and working under simulated sunlight (natural or full-spectrum lighting) have shown a decrease in stress and anxiety, improved behavior and attitudes, improved health and attendance, and increased performance and academic achievement.

Follow the Sun

Benjamin Franklin admonished people to 'Keep in the sunlight.' An old Irish saying put it this way: 'May the sun shine bright on your windowpane.' Find a way to get the amount of light your brain needs. Spend some time outdoors during daylight hours if at all possible, but try to avoid direct sun at high noon and wear your sunglasses. Consider keeping television and other electronics out of your bedroom. Make sure your room is very dark at night. Cover any LED lights that could trigger your melatonin cycle if you awakened during the night. These strategies may enhance your quality of sleep and, consequently, improve your mood and energy levels the next day.

Key factor number eighteen scares some people but it is extremely valuable—used appropriately. Turn to the next chapter.

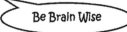

Be Brain Wise

Develop, maintain, nurture, and access your own support network on a regular basis. Select members with care. Choose those who are smart, happy, have a good sense of humor, laugh a lot, and are on a similar high-level-healthiness journey.

Who you hang out with can make a huge difference not only to the quality of your own life but also to your potential longevity. And your lifestyle choices can also influence the lives and choices of others.

Key Factor—18
Support Network

We should look for someone to eat and drink with before looking for something to eat and drink.

—Epicurus

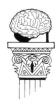 "Welcome to our neighborhood," said Neil, putting out his hand over their common fence. "Glad to meet you. Neighbors can be a great support network for each other."

"Support network?" asked Andy. "We don't need any touchy-feely group of friends. We take care of ourselves."

"Same here," said Neil, smiling. "But John Donne famously said no one is an island, each is a piece of the continent or something to that effect. Neighbors can help watch each other's back: pick up the paper if you're away for the weekend, notice if a water-pipe bursts or a fire ignites."

Andy and Angela had the grace to look a bit embarrassed. "We've never lived in town before, much less next door to anyone. Certainly not to another family," said Angela.

"Support network," said Andy. "That's a new concept, certainly a new label. I find the idea rather intriguing. It would be nice to know that someone *had your back*, as you put it. Thanks." This time Andy put out his hand for a shake.

Relational Brain

The human brain is a relational brain and wired to connect. It is, by design, sociable. Each person needs a personal support network—a core group of individuals with whom to share interests, encouragement, connection, and celebration. Studies have shown a tight inverse relationship between sociability and mortality. Individuals who interact with a nurturing support network of selected individuals generally are healthier and live longer than those who don't.

Dr. Daniel Goleman in his book entitled *Social Intelligence,* points out:

> *Our relationships have subtle, yet powerful, lifelong impacts on us . . . Nourishing relationships have a beneficial impact on our health, while toxic ones can act like slow poison in our bodies . . . Our relationships mold not just our personal experience but also our biology.*

A support network is made up of friends, family, family-of-choice, peers, neighbors, and in some instances even pets. It differs from a support group that is generally a structured meeting facilitated by a health professional and with a specific topic to be discussed.

Although both can play important roles in times of stress, a support network is something you can develop when you're not under stress. In fact, that's the best time to do it, when you don't think you may need it. Those who have a support network tout its benefits and there can be many of them—because no one is an island. At least not successfully.

Benefits

Make the support-network concept work for you. Surround yourself with *pieces of the continent.* The benefits of a support network can include: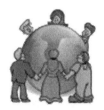

Increased sense of belonging. Whether it's associating with dog lovers, other new moms, fishing buddies, siblings, club members, neighbors, or hobbyists, knowing you're not alone can be immensely helpful.

Increased sense of self-worth. Knowing people who consider you part of their support network—and with whom you reciprocate—reinforces the idea that you're a valuable person to be around. When you also share brain-function similarities, the commonality can help you to feel *smart* when you are with each other.

Increased sense of security. By reaching out and sharing yourself with others, you have the added security of knowing that if you start to show signs of depression or exhibit unhealthy lifestyle habits, your friends can help alert you to the problem.

In *Timeless Healing* author Herbert Benson MD reported on a study of nearly 7,000 men and women between the ages of 30 and 69 in Alameda County, California. Researchers found that social isolation has pervasive negative health consequences. Higher degrees of social connection, on the other hand, consistently related to decreased mortality. George Bernard Shaw put it this way, we are all dependent on one another.

Choose Carefully

In this current culture, often there may be few if any extended family members in close proximity. Therefore, you may need to create a family-of-choice—individuals who are willing to function in the role of family members and who are on your same mental wavelength. Anything that keeps you in healthy contact with others tends to help you live better and longer. Select your friends with care, however. According to motivational speaker Jim Rohn, you are the average of the five people with whom you spend the most time; you being one of them, as you are the only person who will be with you for your entire life. These individuals influence you in many different ways—from your level of cheerfulness, weight, the habits you develop, the behaviors you exhibit (e.g., smoking or not), the goals you set, and the things you think and talk about. Spending time with individuals who are codependent or who are engaged in the same types of unhealthy behaviors that you may be trying to change—whether substance abuse, an addictive behavior, or a negative attitude—can sabotage your personal growth. They directly impact who you are and how you behave.

Studies have shown that within about three years, you tend to mimic the behaviors of those with whom you hang out. If you are in relationships in which you are neither helping yourself nor anybody else, you are likely not being the best you can be and, therefore, not being the best you can be to them, either. This is where the proverbial rubber meets the road. If your friends, family members, or support network do not encourage, affirm, and help you become a better person, you may need to reduce the amount of time spent with them.

And if they are seriously dragging you down, abusing you or encouraging you to abuse yourself (e.g., enabling serious addictive behaviors), you may need to find healthier and more positive replacements. One person framed this in a nutshell: If you and your plus four are positive-minded and believe in taking responsibility for your life, you will tend to become a proactive individual who shapes your future. Conversely, if you and your plus four are pessimistic, think and speak negatively, believe there's very little worthwhile in life, and that others are out to get you so you better get them first, you will tend to swirl down into a negative whirlpool, even if initially you were a more positive person. It may sound hard but your longevity and overall success has a great deal to do with who you select for your family-of-choice, support network, or close friends—whatever terminology works for you.

Three Degrees

Do you remember the concept known as 'six degrees of separation?' It's gotten tighter. Harvard Medical School researchers have identified a *happiness cascade*. Your happiness is most likely to boost the happiness levels in people closest to you: family members, close friends, support network, and co-workers. However, your happiness levels can also spread outward through three degrees of separation and can impact people that you may not even know—and vice versa. Make friends with happy people, those who are smart, have high levels of emotional intelligence, possess a good sense of humor, laugh a lot, and are on your high-level-healthiness journey. Hone those same qualities in yourself, knowing that you are impacting many others.

Studies by Dr. Rosemary Blieszner, professor of human development at Virginia Tech, concluded that people who are surrounded by happy people are more likely to be happy in the future than those who are surrounded by unhappy people. The goal of building a support network is to reduce your stress level, not to add to it. The negative consequences of maintaining 'obligatory' relationships, especially when they are draining and not reciprocal, affirming, and healthy, can far outweigh the benefits. Although you may not choose to completely sever ties with a negative, nagging relative or friend, look for ways of managing the relationship to minimize negative stress to yourself. Perhaps you can connect some of the time by phone, snail mail, or e-mail rather than always face-to-face. Sometimes people hold on to dysfunctional relationships far longer than is good for them. Marc Chernoff put it this way:

You will only ever be as great as the people with whom you surround yourself; so be brave enough to let go of those who keep bringing you down.

The Past is Not an Unalterable Future

Scientists now understand that lifestyle choices are particularly important in terms of the impact to the fetus during gestation. A pregnant mother's choices (e.g., cigarettes, alcohol, level of nutrition, exercise) can have a huge impact on her unborn child. The amount and type of stressors play a part, too. The children of pregnant women who saw the 9-11 World Trade catastrophe were found to have higher levels of cortisol. Posttraumatic Stress Disorder or PTSD may even be transmitted from one generation to the next.

According to Debra Bangasser PhD, a child who experienced a stressful pregnancy may require higher levels of stress just to activate the release of cortisol. Waiting to do things until the very last minute may be indicative of this. For a female fetus, a stressful pregnancy (and/or a stressful first two years of life) can actually result in the female developing a more reactive brain and nervous system, which can increase her reactivity to stress over a lifetime.

It surprises some to find out that their father's habits can impact his children and grandchildren, as well. The ALSPAC study showed that males who started smoking before age 11 (just before entering puberty and before they were producing sperm) influenced the health of their sons. By age nine, their boys had significantly higher body mass indexes (BMI). This considerably increased their risk of obesity and other serious health issues including a shortened lifespan.

Since no one influences what parents and grandparents do or even what happens during their own gestation or for the first few years of life, some may feel hopeless. Nothing could be further from the truth. Potentially you can revolutionize your own health through the lifestyle you choose to live and those with whom you surround yourself. Develop a support network and make thoughtful and careful choices about the members you select. Choose to live a high-level-healthiness lifestyle and create a healthier future for yourself and those you love.

Key factor number nineteen is linked with both gratitude and forgiveness. The next chapter may surprise you.

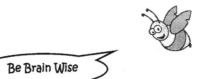

Be Brain Wise

According to Ezra Taft Benson, youth embodies the spirit of adventure and awakening. Carry that perspective with you. Hone your own personal sense of spirit—the way in which you approach and live life.

Regularly engage in activities that trigger a sense of awe within your brain. Do random acts of kindness. Live a forgiving life—of yourself and of others. Start and end each day with gratitude. It's an antidote for fear.

Key Factor—19
Sensible Spirituality

*Hone your spirituality—the spirit in which you live life.
Avoid allowing an unchangeable past or an uncertain
future to ruin the splendid gift of today.*

—Old Saying

 "Our professor told us in class today that although many people consider the concepts of spirituality and religion as basically synonymous, they are in fact quite different," said Alex. "Most of the class thought they were one and the same. I wanted to ask him how they differed but I had to hurry off to my lab assignment. What's your take, Dad?"

"Interesting you should ask," said his father. "I've just finished reading *Why We Believe What We Believe* by Newberg and Waldman. They point out that the human mind may be naturally calibrated to embrace spiritual perceptions. I figure that makes spirituality a sensible topic to investigate."

"Our professor said that defining spirituality can be a challenge because it is very subjective and differs for each brain—and each brain on the planet differs. So guess what?" asked Alex. "Our assignment for next class is to craft our own personal definition. I could probably use a little help with that. Hint, hint," he added, laughing.

"Let's get on our computers and see what we can find out. I'll enjoy doing this with you," said his father.

A few minutes later Alex pointed at his monitor. The two read silently.

- Religion involves a choice to affiliate with specific theologies (rules, rituals, rites, or dogma) that have been endorsed by an organization or denomination.

- Spirituality encompasses the spirit in which you live life, your ethical and moral choices; helping you understand and find purpose and meaning in life; a sense of awe for something greater than yourself; and a vision to achieve the highest possible levels of healthiness and longevity.

"It appears they may be different concepts," said Alex.

"This site says whatever else human brains are, they are relational, sexual, and spiritual," said his father. "A strong spirituality is being linked with a variety of health benefits including lower depression rates and enhanced relationships. Doctor N. Lee Smith, director of the Stress Medicine Clinic at the University of Utah, talks about spiritual health as a state of well-being—not just the absence of disease. That sounds a lot like high-level-healthiness to me. Those who are part of a spiritual community have been shown to have lower blood pressure and a reduced risk of cardiovascular disease, lower rates of suicide, lower rates of substance abuse, and stronger immune systems."

"I'll print off a couple of these references and work on my definition," said Alex. "Thanks, Dad."

A Sense of Awe

Defining spirituality can be a bit challenging. Some have explained it as the sense of awe you experience when overwhelmed with the beauty of nature, music, architecture, religious rites, meditation, or a connection with a Higher Power as you perceive it, or when in the grip of deep compassion, empathy, or gratitude. The triggers for awe in your brain and the choices you make related to spirituality are impacted by a myriad of factors. Some are based on information, education, and expectations, while others involve past experiences, innate giftedness, role-modeling, or personal desire. Some advocate identifying what evokes a sense of awe in your brain and regularly engaging in those experiences.

Benefits of Meditation

Studies have found that meditation or prayer, as a form of meditation, changes your brain. MRI scans have shown that people who meditate regularly show an increase in size in several parts of the brain. They have large frontal lobes where the brain's executive functions are located, they increase the amount of gray matter in the midbrain (that handles functions such as blood circulation and breathing) and in the prefrontal cortex (involved with active memory), and so on. Those who meditate or pray regularly have less brain atrophy. Every brain on the planet is unique, however, so each brain's meditative experience will be different.

Dr. Paul Pearsall pointed out in *The Heart's Code* that virtually every spiritual tradition includes some form of meditation.

Contemplative states, such as that induced by Dr. Stroebel's Quieting Reflex, tend to result in positive physical changes including slower breathing and heart rate, lowered blood pressure, and relaxation of tense muscles. The bodies of runners who meditated or prayed while exercising were found to function more effectively than those who did not.

Brain efficiency can be strengthened by meditation. Owen Felltham, 15th century English poet and essayist, is credited with saying: *Meditation is the soul's perspective glass.* During the quiet contemplation that is typically associated with meditation or prayer, you can begin to view events and life in a new way. Implement a meditation style that works for you. Engage in mindful thanksgiving, since a grateful heart nourishes the brain and spirit. Identify what is positive in your life and concentrate on those aspects.

Universal Scope

Best-selling author Donald E. Sloat PhD has been quoted as saying: 'Our spiritual lives have a foundation in our psychological selves. If we have the idea that there is no connection between the natural (temperament and personality structure) and the supernatural (our spiritual lives), we are seriously mistaken.'

Actor Martin Sheen had an interesting perspective, as well:

The direction of the universe can and will be determined by the presence of individual spirituality or the lack of it. If you would change the world, change yourself and it is done.

Spirituality and Energy

Emerging data point to a connection between spirituality and energy. In her best-selling book *Anatomy of the Spirit,* Dr. Carolyn Myss pointed out:

> *Our bodies thrive when our spirits thrive . . . One's spiritual thoughts and activities are inseparable from other aspects of life . . . From an energy point of view, every choice that enhances our spirits strengthens our energy field.*

M. Scott Peck, author of *The Road Less Traveled* believed that those who are seeking for but unable to find a desired spiritual life, may substitute an addictive behavior for the spiritual connection they crave but cannot develop.

Spirituality-Gratitude Link

Spirituality and gratitude may be linked. In his book *Thanks!* Robert Emmons points out that people who practice grateful thinking reap many emotional, physical, and interpersonal benefits. They tend to take better care of themselves and engage in more protective health behaviors like physical and mental exercise, healthy eating, and regular physical examinations.

Individuals who keep a gratitude journal—hard copy or electronic—report fewer symptoms of illness, tend to feel better about their lives as a whole, and typically are much more hopeful about the future. Gratitude is *good medicine.* Grateful people tend to be more optimistic, a characteristic that researchers say boosts immune system function.

Studies by Martin Seligman point out that individuals who write 'gratitude letters' to a person who made a difference in their lives score higher on happiness, and lower on depression—and the effect lasts for weeks. And, according to Melanie Greenberg PhD, clinical psychologist, life coach, and expert on life change, developing a gratitude practice can open your heart and rewire your brain.

Edward Diener PhD, professor at the University of Illinois at Champaign-Urbana and also known as Dr. Happiness, has studied life satisfaction of people from various cultures. He found, for example, that people in India living in poverty report low levels of life satisfaction. But so do a high percentage of people in affluent Japan. This suggests that an emphasis on materialism may be partially to blame.

Dubbed the 'Queen of All Media,' Oprah Winfrey may be best known for *The Oprah Winfrey Show*. It has been touted as the highest rated program of its kind in history and was nationally syndicated from 1986 to 2011. This is her perspective: 'Be thankful for what you have; you'll end up having more. If you concentrate on what you don't have, you will never, ever have enough.'

Research by David DeSteno at Northeastern University in Boston has shown that gratitude reduces impatience. Although different, gratitude and happiness may actually reinforce each other, positively impacting mindset, self-talk, attitude, and communication. You can move up your set point to some degree for both happiness and gratitude—in all likelihood enough to have a measurable effect on both your overall outlook and health.

Studies at the University of Connecticut found that patients who identified benefits from their heart attack—such as becoming more appreciative of life—lowered their risk of having another heart attack.

You may have heard of the Native American Shawnee Warrior, Tecumtha, often referred to as Tecumseh. A proponent of gratitude, he has been quoted as saying:

> *When you rise in the morning, give thanks for the light, for your life, for your strength. Give thanks for your food and for the joy of living. If you see no reason to give thanks, give thanks anyway.*

A strong spirituality is being linked with a variety of health benefits including lower depression rates, and enhanced relationships. It also appears to be linked with a willingness to forgive. Work by Dr. Herbert Benson has shown many positive health-related outcomes to those who choose to forgive—themselves as well as others. In fact, this appears to be independent of whether or not the person being forgiven even knows about it. Do it for yourself because the one who forgives benefits the most. Make choices that enhance your sense of spirit, increase your wisdom, and generate energy. Live in gratitude and forgiveness. Create a spiritual vision for yourself and take steps to leave this planet a better place than you found it.

The twentieth key factor is up next. Are you able to bend with the storm or do you break? Turn the page and check out the next chapter.

Be Brain Wise

Flexibility is invaluable to growing older successfully— even gracefully—especially in relation to brain function. Innately the brain has a great deal of plasticity. Avoid allowing your mindset to harden and become brittle.

Stay flexible. Imagine yourself as a tree. Picture yourself bending gracefully with the wind and then returning to an upright position.

Key Factor—20
Flexible Plasticity

A tree that is unbending is easily broken.

—Lao Tzu (c. 604 - 531 BCE)

"Granddad," said Lachlan, "I have a question."

Granddad put down the book he was reading and smiled at his grandson. "Fire away."

"Today I heard my teacher talking about the brain. He said it was plastic. What part is plastic?" asked Lachlan.

"Your teacher likely meant *plasticity*," said his Granddad, "unless he was talking about a model of the brain."

"What is plasticity and is it a good thing?" persisted the boy.

"Scientists believe it is not only a good thing but also quite amazing, as well," said Granddad, smiling. "They explain it as the brain's innate ability to be flexible and adaptable and learn new things. It can create new software programs, much as on your computer, and can even rewire itself or its software programs if it or part of the body is injured."

"Oh," said Lachlan. "When Tiger was hit by a car and lost a leg, he learned to walk on only three legs almost as well. Was that plasticity for his brain?"

"It most certainly was," said his Granddad. "The same thing happens in your brain when you learn to ride a two-wheel bicycle, whiz around on your skateboard, nail a new video game, learn to play a new song on your violin, and do a host of other activities that you've not done before. That's the marvelous *plasticity* of your brain. It also helps you to improve your skills for a specific activity like memorizing music on the piano and then dashing it off flawlessly at your recital. It's somewhat of a metaphor, however, because your brain is composed of living cells rather than the *plastic* you're familiar with in the outside world."

"Neurons and all that stuff," said Lachlan, nodding. "Is your brain plastic, too, or just kids' brains?"

"Thankfully, yes," Granddad replied. "Otherwise I'd have been in a world of hurt last year when that tree branch snapped off and broke my right arm in several places." Lachlan nodded. "I had to do everything with my left hand and arm. When the cast was removed after months later, I was nearly ambidextrous. I'd learned to use my left hand and arm almost as well as my right."

"Not at first, Granddad," Lachlan said, laughing. "You poured juice on the table instead of in my glass,"

"I sure did. And the first time I cleaned my teeth by holding the brush in my left hand toothpaste went flying everywhere. Your Grandmother was not amused, as I recall."

"I'd like to teach people how rewire their brain after an injury," said Lachlan. "And write new software for a stellar computer game. I'm very glad to know about plasticity."

"You and cabbies in London," said Granddad. "What researchers have discovered about their brains is really encouraging in terms of life-long learning, especially for those of us who are fortunate enough to keep having birthdays." He laughed. "Studies showed that learning how to navigate the thousands of streets in the bustling and often crowded streets of the London metropolis actually changed the brains of the taxi drivers." Lachlan sat down cross legged on the floor, listening. "In order to become a licensed cab driver in London, trainees must learn at least 25,000 streets along with their complicated layouts and 20,000 landmarks. The whole process takes three to four years, after which they are required to take a series of examinations, which only about half of the trainees pass.

"Researchers took brain scans at the beginning of the study and again at the end. Compared with the first brain pictures, those taken at the end of training showed a significant increase in gray matter in the hippocampus, your brain's search engine that plays an important role in memory and spatial navigation. These changes were only seen in the brains of drivers who qualified as taxi drivers and not in the brains of those who failed to qualify or in a group of non-taxi-driver controls. Talk about brain plasticity!" He paused briefly and then continued. "Not long ago I watched a program on TV where a woman was being interviewed on the occasion of her 105th birthday. The news anchor asked to what she attributed her long life. Sharp as the proverbial tack, the woman responded, 'Good genes and the ability to flex with the times.' That's plasticity, too."

"Thanks, Granddad," said Lachlan, smiling. "I'll practice my violin now and use some of my brain's plasticity."

Bend or Break

In a severe storm, trees that typically survive are those that can sway with catastrophic conditions and still remain firmly rooted. They bend but do not break. According to Chuck Gallozzi, author of over 200 articles on personal development and national champion of a Toastmasters International Speech Contest, flexibility is a very desirable quality. He points out:

> *To be flexible, we must be willing to break from tradition, custom, and habit. We must be willing to question everything. Keep an open mind, but remember gullibility enslaves you to the opinions of others, while skepticism frees you to discover the value or uselessness inherent in the ideas of others . . . Blessed are the mentally flexible for they shall not get bent out of shape.*

Lack of flexibility frequently triggers reactions rather than thoughtful solution-based responses. This type of unattractive (and usually unhelpful) rigidity may be seen in a variety of oppressive regimes—countries, organizations, and even family systems.

Be very clear that the ability to be flexible by no means implies that you are a wishy-washy person without your own opinions, beliefs, standards, or boundaries. In today's world, with its fast-changing pace and ever-increasing types of technologies, flexibility is essential for your own welfare. It's critical for the overall welfare of humanity and the planet, as well.

Thanks to brain plasticity, mental flexibility allows you to:

- Adapt to change fairly easily and not be thrown off
- Brainstorm solutions to problems
- See multiple perspectives
- Tolerate some uncertainty and ambiguity
- Take calculated risks
- Think practically as well as innovatively

A Dozen Tips

1. Realize that every brain is unique—yours included. All each brain has is *its own opinion* based on its own structure, function, and perception (education, life experiences, expectations, brainwashing, etc.). Some think their opinion is "the only correct one," and it may be in reality, but it's still their brain's opinion.

2. Avoid foolish controversy and meaningless argument. When people argue, at least one of the brains usually 'thinks it really knows' and believes that if it speaks louder and longer, adds some pejoratives, or applies coercion, 'maybe, just maybe that other brain will get it.' Think again!

3. When exposed to the opinions of others, notice ways in which their opinions have impacted their lives, rather than focusing exclusively on how their opinions differ from yours. If their lives have been impacted for the better, avoid dismissing their opinions just because they are new to you or you disagree. You may be able to use part of what you hear or apply it in a new way.

4. Slow down and avoid rushing to disagree (or agree) with another's viewpoint. It's only their brain's opinion and may have nothing to do with yours. However, the more ideas and ways of looking at the same thing to which your brain is exposed the more potential solutions you may have at your fingertips.

5. Remember that some of the most amazing solutions in life come to fruition collectively. Meaning, it often takes a combination of brains contributing their own opinions and giftedness to finally craft something that will work optimally for the majority. Contribute rather than coerce. Realize that no one brain knows everything.

6. Learn from as many different sources as you possibly can. In this 21st century with the world-wide web, there are a plethora of resources available. Learning something new gives you more options to consider, and more options provide additional flexibility.

7. When considering the opinions of others, use your whole brain—the sequential verbal left hemisphere as well as the intuitive creative right hemisphere. Each has valuable gifts to offer. Together they can result in enhanced decision making.

8. Learn to separate the content of another's opinion from the manner in which the opinion was presented. Some brains will be on your wavelength; others will not. If you get sidetracked by the presentation style or the wavelength similarities or differences, you may overlook something valuable.

9. When you perceive discomfort based on the opinions of others, take a deep breath, step back, and accept it as something for you to explore. Sometimes it is because the opinion cuts cross-grain against something you were taught to believe earlier in life. Perhaps their opinions have brought to the surface some belief or attitude you have absorbed subconsciously and never identified.

10. Hone and access your Emotional Intelligence (EQ) carefully. Avoid JOT behaviors: Jumping to conclusions, Overreacting, or Taking things personally. Bring intelligence to your emotion and emotion to your intelligence. You need the combination. Each provides you with different types of information. Relying on only one or the other gives you only half the potential package and you'll do better with a whole-brain approach.

11. Expect the unexpected. Learn to roll with the punches when something occurs over which you have no control. Stuff happens. If you accept that anything can happen at any time, you're less likely to be thrown off your stride when it does. Collaborate with your brain's plasticity. Hone your flexibility. Be able to adjust your game plan.

12. When struggling with a problem, ask yourself how it might look to someone of another gender, age, career path, political party, race, religion, culture, or socio-economic status. Or pretend you are in an active debate with yourself. State first one position, then advocate for the other. You may be amazed at the insights you gain.

The last key factor, number twenty-one, is next.

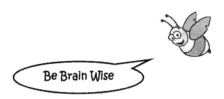

Be Brain Wise

The brain works best when it and your body are humming along in a state of equilibrium, equipoise, balance. Bona fide balance is a key component of high-level-healthiness living.

Aim for real and consistent balance in life, essential for health, happiness, success, and longevity. Learn to manage your swings and keep them in as balanced a range as possible.

Key Factor—21
Bona Fide Balance

Live a balanced life—learn some and think some and draw some and paint some and sing and dance and play and work every day some.

—Robert Fulghum
All I Really Need to Know I Learned in Kindergarten

 Alana stood in front of the antique grandfather clock in the front hall. "Something is not working right—again," she called to her husband. "This clock is not keeping good time. It ticks for a while and then it stops for a while and then it starts ticking again. But now it's behind the correct time. Very unhelpful in a clock. Matter of fact I see little point in even having an antique grandfather clock if it isn't keeping good time!"

Wayne came and stood beside her. "It's unbalanced again for some reason," he said. "I wonder if the small earthquakes we've been having in the region are impacting it. I'll call the clock-maker and ask him to send his seventy-year-old assistant out to rebalance it. He's getting up there."

"Pooh," said Alana. "That's nothing compared to Jeanne Louise Calment's longevity of 122 years 164 days."

Wayne smiled and shrugged. "Nevertheless . . ."

Later at breakfast Alana said, "I feel a little like our antique grandfather clock—out of balance. My life isn't working very well right now, especially since I took that new job two years ago. Managing a department is not my cup of tea. I was much happier managing a program."

"Is your old job available?" asked Wayne. "There wasn't all that much difference in salary and I've been concerned about you for months. I expected there'd be some additional stress at first but you are always tired and seem really unhappy. I'd like my old Alana back and I'll bet your brain would, too."

"You're right. I don't love this job and my life is out of balance. I'm not even sure what a balanced life looks like anymore," said Alana.

"To me it means you have a handle on the various elements in your life and don't sense that your brain and your heart are in a tug of war," said Wayne. "Typically you're motivated, think clearly, and are calmly grounded in reality, and enjoying most if not all aspects of your life."

Alana sat very still for a long moment. Finally she said, "I'll stop in at Human Resources this morning. Returning to my old job just might be a viable possibility. Thank you, Wayne."

"Good," said her husband. "I think you're close to burnout and life isn't worth that."

With a hug and a kiss, they were out the door. Wayne, noticing that his wife had a spring in her step for the first time since she had taken that new job, smiled.

Brain and Balance

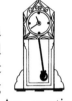

Likely you've seen the pendulum of a grandfather clock swinging back and forth and back and forth. It can be comforting, almost hypnotic. A pendulum that has stopped swinging means the clock has stopped functioning. An erratic pendulum tends to wobble, swing wildly from side to side, or crash into the glass and stop. Much like a well-running grandfather clock, the brain works best in balance—when everything is working congruently. Thomas Merton said that happiness is not a matter of intensity but of balance, order, rhythm, and harmony. Balance can be hard to find. Nevertheless, it's a goal worth pursuing.

According to Daniel G. Amen MD, author of *Magnificent Mind at any Age,* a magnificent mind begins with a balanced brain. A state of imbalance can leave your brain fatigued, discouraged, irritated, and screaming for relief. This can put you at increased risk for any number of brain dysfunctions, illnesses, or disease. You and your brain must identify your own priorities and find your own balance.

Life is constantly changing so finding balance is somewhat of a moving target. What is right for you now may not be right next week or next month or even next year, because priorities change over time. If you are struggling with 'where the times goes,' jot down for a few days what you are spending your time doing. This will help you identify and evaluate whether you're allocating your time in the most productive or desirable way—based on your personal and professional goals. You may need to re-evaluate those goals. Some may no longer be realistic or even desirable.

Boundaries

Some have referred to balance as the ultimate goal. That may not be far off. But balance and boundaries are twins, Siamese twins. In her book *A Life in Balance* Dr. Kathleen A. Hall wrote: 'We have overstretched our personal boundaries and forgotten that true happiness comes from 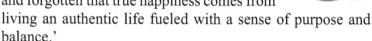 living an authentic life fueled with a sense of purpose and balance.'

Evaluate your mental, emotional, physical, sexual, social, financial, educational, spiritual, and romantic boundaries, to name just a few. Are they too tight, too loose, nonexistent, or just right for you and a high-level healthiness lifestyle? Developing and implementing bona fide boundaries can help you keep your life in bona fide balance. Your boundaries are as individual as your brain and your thumbprint, and your daily choices impact everything. Even not making a decision is a type of decision. This is especially true when it comes to understanding how to age-proof your brain. You can only do what you know. Evaluate what needs to be tweaked and begin making desirable lifestyle changes a little at a time. That way your improvements will be more likely to last!

Burnout

Burnout is a state of mental, emotional, and physical exhaustion caused by excessive and prolonged stress. It triggers a sense of being overwhelmed from being unable to meet all the constant demands made of you. Burnout leads to lowered energy levels, fatigue and exhaustion, and can push you to be reactive rather than proactive.

As your self-confidence and enjoyment in life collapse, so can your health and well-being, to say nothing of your relationships and goals. Those who crash and burn are often those who think they are super-heroes who can and must do everything and do it flawlessly. No such people really exist in the long term—except on paper and in cartoon series. Many think that living in balance means spending the same amount of time on each segment of life that is important to you. Big mistake. Some areas need more time than others, some less. The problem arises when you neglect important areas of life, which if not balanced will negatively influence your ability to be successful and happy: sleep, exercise, good nutrition, fun and play, quality time with family and friends—and with yourself to think and envision.

It's no longer life as your grandparents knew it. You live on a planet that is now frantic with technologies. Some are helpful; some aren't. Your brain is exposed to and receives thousands of times more information and stimuli than brains received only a scant generation ago. Unless you are vigilant, the ever-increasing stimuli your brain receives can push its functions off balance. It has been said that if you love what you do, you will never work a day in your life. Yeah, maybe, but only if you keep your life in balance. If you don't, you may end up hating what you once loved. No one is immune to burnout. It can creep up on you stealthily, especially when you keep adding tasks and activities without dropping others. Live in balance. Down the line that can help you avoid lamenting that you forgot to 'smell the roses' or failed to spend quality time with good friends and family, or spent way too much time on the job.

Get in Balance

Awareness is the first step on the ladder of positive change. You can only manage what you can bring to conscious awareness, label, and describe. Become more aware of the way you are living your life and whether or not it is in balance. You can help prevent burnout or get back in balance by looking at the big picture and deciding what is most important at this stage of your life. Set your priorities and stick to them by working smarter and not harder, by saying 'no' when you have reached your capacity (and know what that is). An increase in conscious awareness could pay huge dividends to enhance your health, wellbeing, and balance. When something new comes into your life (a baby, hobby, or friend) be willing and proactive about giving something up (e.g., a museum-quality home environment, or doing all the house and yard work yourself).

You can take charge of your life and pull your own strings, or you can allow yourself to be manipulated like a puppet. Pulling your own strings is the best way to stay in balance. The brain works best in balance. Period. But it can only do what it thinks it can do and your attitude, thoughts, and self-talk convey to it what it can do. Following are some things to consider.

- Simplify and stop trying to keep up with anyone else— it's your life, your energy, and your longevity

- Shut off all electronics an hour before bedtime (unless you must specifically be 'on call'); get the television out of your bedroom

- Let your phone go to voice mail during mealtimes; disable work email when on holiday

- Be intentional and balanced about social media—avoid allowing it to eat up valuable time every day

- Stop majoring in minors. Identify what is major and focus on that. Let the rest, the minor stuff, go.

- Destress with brain breathing, the Quieting Reflex, meditation, music, or other strategy that works for your brain and body

- Get your mindset, attitude, and self-talk in line to maximize your available energy

- Take time to reflect, play, and have fun—life goes by faster than you might think

Remember the 20:80 Rule? Living the 20:80 Rule can help you avoid giant pendulum swings that push you from one extreme to the other. Not only can it help you minimize negative consequences to your brain and body from stressors, but it can also help you keep a balanced perspective when confronted with the slings and arrows of outrageous fortune. Allow it to enable you to laugh at the vagaries of life—with a sense of humor and style all your own—and thrive by design.

There's one more chapter. The last chapter. It's a bonus that challenges you to *Reach for 122*. Turn the page.

Be Brain Wise

Actively embrace high-level-healthiness living. Set your goals, do something every day to move you closer to them.

Get going!

It's a journey.

As Will Rogers put it, "Even if you are on the right track, you'll get run over if you just sit there."

Reach for 122

Seventy percent of how long and how well you live is in your hands.

—Michael F. Roisen MD and Mehmet C. Oz MD

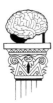 "I'd like to live a long time," said Mary, walking along beside her neighbor. "My parents both died well before the age of seventy and that seems such a short lifetime from my perspective of eighty-four."

"I agree," said Martha. "And I, for one, like the new information that is coming out about how long human beings really can live. I am aiming higher."

"How high are you aiming?" asked Mary. "You know I want to live to at least age ninety."

"I'm aiming higher than that," said Martha, laughing.

"Higher than ninety?" asked Mary. "How much higher?"

"More than a quarter of a century higher," replied Martha, seriously. "I'm aiming for 122 years 164 days. That's how old Jeanne Louise Calment was when she died in 1997. She was born in Arles, Southern France, in 1875 and lived there her whole life. That unflappable woman took up fencing at age eighty-five and rode her bicycle until she was age one hundred! I'd say her life demonstrates the old adage, *you'll get farther if you aim higher.*"

"Oh, my goodness!" exclaimed Mary. "Where did you hear about her?"

"On National Public Radio," said Martha. "Club 122 Longevity was named for her. There's even a website for people who are aiming higher, who are learning about how to live younger longer through creating and maintaining a Longevity Lifestyle: www.LongevityLifestyleMatters.com.

"I just revised my personal goal," said Mary, laughing. "I'm aiming to be at least 122 years 164 days. If Jeanne Louise Calment could do it, so can I!"

Aim High

According to Marilyn Ferguson, author of *Aquarius Now,* of all the self-fulfilling prophecies in our culture, the assumption that aging means decline and poor health is probably the deadliest. Unfortunately, many people have bought into that perspective. You can make a different choice. Aiming to be a centenarian and beyond is no longer just pie-in-the-sky wishful thinking. You may be one of those who live that long. Either way, Martha was correct: you'll get farther if you aim higher.

Ronald Klatz MD, and Robert Goldman MD, authors of *The Anti-Aging Revolution,* put it this way:

> *The reality for 76 million Baby Boomers will be an average life span in excess of 100 years, with unexpectedly good health—so much so, in fact, that you will scarcely be able to tell a fit and active 65-year old from a healthy and athletic 105-year-old.*

170

Cicero reportedly said that old age must be resisted and its deficiencies supplied. Fortunately, studies on aging are providing insight into how to die young at a very old age—or how to live younger longer, if you like that wording better. That perspective is something many people could get excited about doing; could jump on board wholeheartedly.

Can you control all the factors that impact aging and the brain? No. Can you impact many of them? Yes! Estimates are that more than half the factors that have been found to impact the process of growing older are within your partial, if not complete, control. Identify those factors in your life and take responsibility for them. Put your time, energy, and money into those.

Sure heredity plays a part. However, emerging perspectives are that 70 percent of how long you live and how well you live is in your hands. The most effective strategies for preserving brain function and preventing decline (insofar as it is possible to do so) involve components of high-level-healthiness living. A well-functioning body without a sound brain doesn't get you very far.

A lifestyle that leads to healthy longevity involves an approach that emphasizes more than the absence of disease and goes beyond what is often considered to be 'normal' levels of health. After all, the word normal simply means commonly occurring. Something that occurs commonly may be neither desirable nor healthy. This is true about the process of growing older, as well, in general and brain health in particular.

Safety First

Since everything starts in the brain, it is vitally important to protect it—you only have one and so far it's irreplaceable. Think ahead and be proactive. Head injuries can alter your life significantly because brain tissue is very soft, as soft as room-temperature butter. Consider the following prevention strategies to help protect your brain.

- Always wear your seat belt in vehicles
- Avoid contact sports
- Wear sturdy shoes to prevent slipping
- Avoid scatter rugs that might trip you up
- Wear a helmet when biking
- Swim with a friend, never alone
- Wear head protection when engaged in any activity that might result in a fall or injury
- Pay attention and be aware—distracted walking can lead to falls and head injuries
- Eat breakfast. According to Pediatrician Bill Sears MD, eating breakfast is critical for your brain. It restocks the energy stores that have been depleted overnight. Without breakfast, you may lose up to 40 percent of your energy efficiency by noon.

Avoid or minimize your exposure to toxic substances that can negatively impact brain function, such as:

- Environmental toxins and pesticides
- Tobacco smoke or side-stream smoke
- Poor quality air
- Alcohol and other drugs, legal or street, as well as excessive over-the-counter medications

An old proverb says, if you continue to do what you've always done, you'll continue to get what you've always gotten. What have you gotten so far in life? Is it what you want to get for the rest of your life?

As Dr. George E Guthrie wrote in the Foreword to *Longevity Lifestyle Matters:*

> *For your health to actually improve, something needs to change. Your healthcare professional can help to guide you with wise use of technology but you will be the one most responsible for changing your lifestyle.*

What does that really mean? For one thing, it means that in order to live a long time with high levels of mental, emotional, physical, and spiritual function, in all likelihood you will need to make some changes in how you are living. It also means that making healthier choices each day are of primary importance in restoring health that has been lost. Lost, often, due to poor lifestyle practices.

Everyone faces challenges, often involving level of health, chronic illness, dementia, and potential longevity. As James Arthur Baldwin put it:

> *Not everything that is faced can be changed—but nothing can be changed until it is faced.*

What are you facing? What needs to be improved? Identify what needs improving because you can deal effectively only with what you can label and describe. Then get started taking steps to improve, one at a time.

Aim higher to get farther. Tell your brain that you are a centenarian in process! Is this really possible, you may ask? Current research suggests that the answer is *yes*. Scientists are explaining not only that this is possible but also how to make it happen.

> You control how healthy you are . . . and how long you are going to live . . . there is no biological reason why we cannot live to be over age 100.
> —Dr. Robert Willix Jr.

> Because the mind influences every cell in the body, human aging is fluid and changeable; it can speed up, slow down, stop for a time and even reverse itself. —Deepak Chopra MD

What really is healthy aging? How's this for a definition:

Healthy aging is the slowest possible rate at which you can die while still maintaining high levels of mental, emotional, physical, social, and spiritual health.

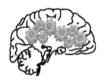 This is the age of the brain. Researchers now know more about how the brain functions than at any other time in the history of our world. That's exciting!

Although there are no magic fixes, research has demonstrated doable strategies that can help you age-proof your brain and reduce your risk for obesity, heart disease, diabetes type 2, dementia, cancers, and other undesirable conditions—which may also increase your longevity.

There has never been another brain just like yours on this planet nor will there ever be again. Although there is no *one size fits all*, studies have identified general principles of 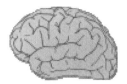 health and longevity that can apply to every individual in some way and help you take good care of your unique brain. The goal is to live a lot of years while keeping life in those years. Apply principles of high-level-healthiness living in ways that work for you and maintain them for your entire sojourn on this planet.

You have nearly reached the end of this book. Hopefully you are grateful for the opportunity to grow older. Also, hopefully, you are excited about what you can do to not only live a long time but also keep life in your years.

Sanford Graves' perspective is that people don't grow old. When they stop growing they become old. According to the Talmud, old age is winter for the unlearned but for the learned it is the season of harvest. Keep learning and growing. Role-model high-level-healthiness living that is helping you age-proof your brain.

May everything and everyone you touch be just a little bit better for having crossed paths with you and your marvelous brain.

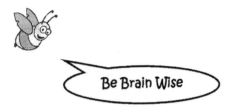

Be Brain Wise

Knowledge is power. People perish every day due to the lack of it. Do something every day to increase what you know about the brain.

Until it is applied, however, information is just a collection of facts. Take the information you learn, turn it into knowledge, and practically apply it on a daily basis.

Authors & Resources

Everything begins in your brain, including your health and potential longevity.
—Sharlet M. Briggs

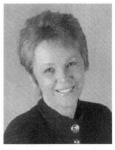 Sharlet M. Briggs PhD, a sought-after speaker, mentor, and author, has an infectious this-can-be-done-and-it's-not-as-hard-as-you-think attitude. This is coupled with an ability to empower individuals to change their perception and as a result, change their realities.

Briggs speaks internationally, sharing brain-function and healthcare information in a practical, engaging, and enlightening style.

Briggs is Chief Operating Officer at a large healthcare facility in California. In addition she enjoys educating adults, youth, and children about the brain and brain function.

She has authored and co-authored books and DVD's.

Briggs has an earned doctorate in Clinical Psychology.

Contact Dr. Briggs at: www.SharletBriggs.com
www.LLM.life
www.LongevityLifestyleMatters.com

Books and audiobooks by the Authors

- *Age-Proofing Your Brain—21 Factors You Can Control, 2nd Edition* (hardcopy, audiobook)

- *Age-Proofing Your Memory, four versions* (hardcopy)

- *Longevity Lifestyle Matters—Keeping Your Brain, Body, and Weight in the Game* and the *Companion Notebook* (hardcopy, audiobook)

- *Adventures of Aimi* (hardcopy, audiobook)

- *Adventures of Stella* (hardcopy, audiobook)

- *Adventures of the Longevity Mystery Club* (hardcopy, audiobook)

- *Chronicles of the Alabaster Owl* (hardcopy, audiobook)

- *Chronicles of the Littlest Dolphin* (hardcopy, audiobook)

- *Chronicles of the Jungle King* (hardcopy, audiobook)

- *Beyond the House of Silence* (hardcopy)

- *Brain Benders - brain aerobic exercises* (hardcopy)

- *Your Brain Has a Bent (Not a Dent) 3rd Edition* (hardcopy, audiobook)

Hardcopies and audiobooks are available through PHEC: pacifichealth.org/store/
Hardcopies and DVDs available through: Amazon.com

You only get one brain and one body to last your entire lifetime. Do everything you can–by design—to keep them functioning at peak performance.
—Arlene R. Taylor

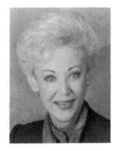 Arlene R. Taylor PhD, an internationally known author and speaker on brain function, is sometimes referred to as the brain guru. A sought-after speaker, she has spoken to thousands internationally, presenting practical brain function information in entertaining, educational, and empowering ways.

Taylor is founder and president of Realizations Inc., a non-profit corporation that engages in brain function research and provides related educational resources. A member of the National Speakers Association and listed with the Professional Speakers Bureau International and Zippii.Com, Taylor has two earned doctorates. Sign up at her website to receive her free quarterly online Brain Bulletin: SynapSez®

Follow Taylor's weekday blog and stimulate your brain while learning more brain bits. Access Taylor's blog from the website homepage (www.arlenetaylor.org), from her Facebook page, or have it sent directly to your email. Remember to 'like' her new Facebook page at:
Arlene R. Taylor PhD Brain Function Specialist.

Contact Dr. Taylor at: www.ArleneTaylor.org
www.LongevityLifestyleMatters.com

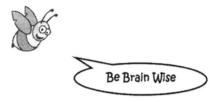

Be Brain Wise

Take advantage of available resources to help you age-proof your brain. Study brain-function information until it becomes an integral part of your knowledge base. Then practically apply what you learn, consistently

Incorporate these key strategies into your high-level-healthiness lifestyle on a daily basis.

Your brain will thank you. So will everyone who knows you!

Selected Bibliography

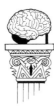 Amen, Daniel G., MD. *Change Your Brain Change Your Life.* NY:Harmony Books, 2015.

_____. *Magnificent Mind at Any Age - Natural Ways to Unleash Your Brain's Maximum Potential.* NY:Harmony Books, 2008.

Appleton, Nancy, PhD. *Lick the Sugar Habit.* NY:Avery Penguin Putnam, 1996.

Batmanghelidjh, Fereydoon, MD. *Your Body's Many Cries for Water*, 3rd Edition. VA:Global Health Solutions, Inc.; 2008.

Batmanghelidjh, Fereydoon, MD. *Water: For Health, for Healing, for Life.* NY:Grand Central Publishing, 2003.

Beck, Martha, PhD. *The Joy Diet.* NY:Crown Publishers, 2003.

Bell, Lynne, and Charlotte Martin. 'The Acute Effects of Low and High doses of Blueberry Flavonoids on Vision, Cognition, and Mood.' (Accessed Nov, 2015) www.reading.ac.uk/psychology/pcls-project-bellmartin.aspx

Benson, Herbert, MD., with Marg Stark. *Timeless Healing: the Power and Biology of Belief.* NY:Scribner, 1996.

Benson, Herbert, MD, with Miriam Z. Klipper. *The Relaxation Response.* NY:Avon Books, 1975.

Benson, Herbert, MD, with William Proctor. *Your Maximum Mind.* NY:Avon Books, 1987.

Boeckner, Linda, and Kay McKinzie. *"Water: The Nutrient."* (Accessed Oct '14) http://www.ianrpubs.unl.edu/epublic/live/g918/build/

Bortz, Water M. II, MD. *We Live Too Short and Die Too Long.* NY:Select Books, 2007.

Bost, Brent W., MD, FACOG. *Hurried Woman Syndrome.* NY:Vantage Press, 2001.

Bragdon, Allen D., and David Gamon, PhD. *Brains that Work a Little Bit Differently.* NY:Barnes and Noble Books, 2000.

Brand-Miller, Jennie, PhD, Thomas M. S. Wolever, MD, PhD, et al. *The New Glucose Revolution.* NY:Marlowe & Company, 2003.

Brmanghelidj F. *Your Body's Many Cries for Water.* VA:Global Health Solutions, 1992.

Broadwell, Richard D., Editor. *Neuroscience, Memory and Language Decade of the Brain, Vol 1.* DC:Library of Congress, 1995.

Brooks, Robert, PhD, and Sam Goldstein, PhD. *The Power of Resilience.* NY:Contemporary Books, McGraw Hill, 2004.

Brynie, Faith Hickman. *101 Questions Your Brain Has Asked About Itself But Couldn't Answer, Until Now.* CT:Millbrook Press, 1998.

Carper, Jean. *Your Miracle Brain.* NY:HarperCollins Publishers, 2000.

Carter, Rita, Ed. *Exploring Consciousness.* CA:University of California Press, 1998.

Carter, Rita, Ed. *Mapping the Mind.* CA:University of California Press, 1998.

Childre, Doc Lew. *Freeze Frame - One Minute Stress Management.* CA:Planetary Publications, 1994, 1998.

Childre, Doc Lew, Howard Martin, Donna Beech, and Institute of HeartMath. *The HeartMath Solution: The Institute of HeartMath's Revolutionary Program for Engaging the Power of the Heart's Intelligence.* NY:HarperOne, 2000.

Chopra, Deepak, MD. *Ageless Body, Timeless Mind.* NY:Harmony Books, 1993.

Cohen, Mark Francis. *What's Worse Than Sugar?* AARP Bulletin, April 2004.

Concoby, Roberts, and David Nicol. *Discovered: Nature's Secret Fountains of Youth.* US:Hanford Press, 1993.

Csikszentmihalyi, Mihaly. *Flow. The Psychology of Optimal Experience.* NY:Harper & Row, 1990.

Deahl, Thomas, D.M.D., PhD. *Water, Thirst, & Dehydration.* CA: Institute for Natural Resources, Health Update. 2009.

Dean, Ward, M.D., and John Morgenthaler and Steven Wm. Fowkes. *Smart Drugs II,* Melatonin Chapter. CA:Smart Publications, 2000.

Dement, William C., MD, PhD, and Christopher Vaughan. *The Promise of Sleep: A Pioneer in Sleep Medicine Explores the Vital Connection Between Health, Happiness, and a Good Night's Sleep.* NY:Dell, 2000.

Diamond, Marian, PhD, and Janet Hopson. *Magic Trees of the Mind.* NY:A Dutton Book, 1998.

Doidge, Norman, MD. *The Brain that Changes Itself.* NY:Penguin Books, 2007.

Dossey, Larry, MD. *Be Careful What You Pray For.* CA:HarperSan Francisco, 1998.

Dossey, Larry, MD. *Healing Words.* NY:Harper Paperbacks, 1993.

Dossey, Larry, MD *Prayer is Good Medicine.* NY:HarperCollins Publishers, 1996.

Douglas, Paul. *Restless Skies: The Ultimate Weather Book.* NY:Sterling, 2007.

Dychtwald, Ken, PhD, and Joe Flo.wer. *Age Wave.* NY:St. Martin's Press, 1989.

Dyer, Wayne, W., PhD. *The Power of Intention.* CA:Hay House, Inc, 2004.

Edell, Dean, MD. *Eat, Drink & Be Merry.* NY:HarperCollins, 1999.

Einberger, Kirstin, and Sellick Janelle, MS. *Strengthen Your Mind.* MD:Health Professions Press, 2007.

Fats (Accessed Jun '16)

   https://www.nlm.nih.gov/medlineplus/ency/patientinstructions/000104.htm

Fisher, Helen, PhD. *Why We Love.* NY:Henry Holt and Company, 2004.

Fontana, David, PhD. *Teach Yourself to Dream: A Practical Guide.* San Francisco, CA:Chronicle Books, 1997.

Fox, Arnold, MD, and Barry Fox, PhD. *Wake Up! You're Alive!* FL:Health Communications, 1988.

Franz, Mary. "Your Brain on Blueberries: Enhance Memory with the Right Foods." Scientific American MIND. January 1, 2011. http://www.scientificamerican.com/article/your-brain-on-blueberries/

Friedman, Edwin H. *What Are You Going to Do with Your Life?* NY:Seabury Books, 2009.

Friedman, Howard S., PhD, and Leslie R. Martin, PhD. *The Longevity Project. Surprising Discoveries for Health and Long Life from the Landmark Eight-Decade Study.* NY:Hudson Street Press, 2011.

Goldberg, Elkhonon. *The Executive Brain.* NY:Oxford University Press, 2001.

Goleman, Daniel, PhD. *Emotional Intelligence.* NY:Bantam Books, 1995.

_____. *Social Intelligence.* NY:Bantam Dell, 2006.

_____. *Working with Emotional Intelligence* NY: Bantam Books, 1998.

Goleman, Daniel, PhD, with Richard Boyatzis, and Annie Mckee. *Primal Leadership.* Boston: Harvard Business School Press, 2002.

Gordon, Barry, MD PhD, and Lisa Berger. *Intelligent Memory.* NY:Penguin Group, 2003.

Giuffre, Kenneth, MD, and Theresa Foy DiGeronimo. *The Care and Feeding of Your Brain: How Diet and Environment Affect What You Think and Feel.* NJ: Career Press Inc, 1999.

Greenwood-Robinson, Maggie, PhD. *20 / 20 Thinking.* NY:Avery, Putnam Special Markets, 2003.

Gurian, Michael, PhD. *From Boys to Men.* NY:Price Stern Sloan, Inc, 1999.

Gurian, Michael, PhD, and Patricia Henley, with Terry Trueman. *Boys and Girls Learn Differently!* CA:Jossey-Bass, 2001.

Gurian, Michael, PhD, and Barbara Annis. *Leadership and the Sexes.* CA:Jossey-Bass, 2008.

Jensen, Anabel L., PhD, et al. *Handle With Care: Emotional Intelligence Activity Book.* CA:Six Seconds, 1998.

Hall, Kathleen A., PhD. *A Life in Balance: Nourishing the Four Roots of True Happiness.* NY:AMACOM, 2006.

Hartmann, Thom. *The Edison Gene.* VT: Park Street Press, 2003.

Healy, Jane M., PhD. *Endangered Minds.* NY:Simon & Schuster, 1990.

Hafen, Brent Q., et al. *Mind/Body Health.* MA:Simon & Schuster, 1996.

Herrmann, Ned. *The Whole Brain Business Book.* NY:McGraw-Hill, 1996.

Howard, Pierce J., PhD. *The Owner's Manual for the Brain. Everyday Applications from Mind-Brain Research.* GA:Bard Press, 1994, 2000.

Jhon, Mu Shik, PhD. *The Water Puzzle and the Hexagonal Key.* UT:Uplifting Press, Inc., 2004. (Translated from Korean by M. J. Pangman.)

Kaiser, Jon D., MD. *Immune Power.* NY:St. Martin's Press, 1993.

Katz, Lawrence C., PhD and Manning Rubin. *Keep Your Brain Alive - 83 Neurobic Exercises to Help Prevent Memory Loss and Increase Mental Fitness.* NY:Workman Publishing Company, Inc., 1999.

Lavizzo-Mourey, Risa J. "Dehydration in the Elderly: A Short Review." http://www.ncbi.nlm.nih.gov/pmc/articles/PMC2625510/)

LeDoux, Joseph. *Synaptic Se lf.* NY:Penguin Books, 2002.

Lazarus, Richard S., PhD. *Stress and Emotion: A New Synthesis.* NY:Springer, 2006.

Levine, Mel, MD. *A Mind at a Time.* NY:Simon & Schuster, 2002.

Lin, James C., Editor. *Advances in Electromagnetic Fields in Living Systems, Volume 2.* (Chapter 1 by Russel J. Reiter.) NY:Springer, 1997.

Lipton, Bruce, PhD. *The Biology of Belief.* CA:Mountain of Love/Elite Books, 2005.

Lombard, Jay, Dr., and Dr. Christian Renna. *Balance Your Brain, Balance Your life.* NJ:John Wiley & Sons, Inc, 2004.

McGraw, Phillip C., PhD. *Self Matters, Creating Your Life From the Inside Out.* NY:Simon & Schuster Source, 2001.

Matthews, Dale, MD, with Connie Clark. *The Faith Factor.* NY:Penguin Books, 1998.

Maas, James B., PhD. *Power Sleep: The Revolutionary Program That Prepares Your Mind for Peak Performance.* NY:Collins Living, 1998.
Mattson, Mark P., PhD. *Diet-Brain Connections: Impact on Memory, Mood, Aging and Disease.* NY:Springer, 2002.

Medina, John. *Brain Rules. 12 Principles for Surviving and Thriving at Work, Home, and School.* WA:Pear Press, 2008.

Merzenich, Michael, PhD. *Soft-Wired: How the new Science of Brain Plasticity Can Change Your Life.* 2nd Edition. CA:Parnassus Publishing, 2013.

Myss, Caroline, PhD. *Anatomy of the Spirit: The Seven Stages of Power and Healing.* NY:Three Rivers Press, 1997.

Nedley, Neil, MD, and edited by David DeRose MD. *Proof Positive – How to Reliably Combat Disease and Achieve Optimal Health through Nutrition and Lifestyle.* OK:Nedley, 1998, 1999.

Neugarten, Bernice L. *The Meanings of Age.* Selected Papers. MI:University of Chicago Press, 1996.

Newberg, Andrew, MD, et al. *Why God Won't Go Away.* NY:Ballantine Books, 2001.

Newberg, Andrew, MD, and Mark Robert Waldman. *Why We Believe What We Believe.* NY:Free Press, 2006.

O'Brien, Mary, MD. *Successful Aging.* CA:Biomed General, 2007.

Oren, Dan A., Editor. *How to Beat Jet Lag.* NY:Holt, 1993.

Ornstein, Robert, PhD. *The Roots of the Self.* NY:HarperCollins Publishing, 1995.

Ornstein, Robert, PhD, and David Sobel, MD. *Healthy Pleasures.* NY:Addison-Wesley, 1990.

Ornstein, Robert, PhD, and Paul Ehrlich. *New World New Mind.* MA:Malor Books, 1989, 2000.

Pearsall, Paul, PhD. *The Heart's Code.* NY:Broadway Books, 1998.

Peck, M. Scott, MD. *People of the Lie: The Hope for Healing Human Evil.* NY:Touchstone, 1998.

_____. *The Road Less Traveled, 25th Anniversary Edition: A New Psychology of Love, Traditional Values and Spiritual Growth.* NY:Touchstone, 2003.

Perricone, Nicholas, MD. *The Perricone Promise.* NY:Warner Books, 2004.

Pert, Candace, B., PhD, and Nancy Marriott. *Everything You Need to Know to Feel Go(o)d.* CA:Hayhouse, 2007.

Pert, Candace, B., PhD. *To Feel Good: The Science and Spirit of Bliss* (Audiobook). CO:Sounds True Inc., 2007.

_____. *Your Body is Your Subconscious Mind* (Audiobook). CO:Sounds True Inc., 2000.

_____. *Molecules of Emotion.* NY:Scribner, 1997.

Pratt, Steven G., and Kathy Mattthews, with Michel Stroot (contributor). *SuperFoods Rx: Fourteen Foods That Will Change Your Life.* NY:Harper, 2006.

Quartz, Steven R., PhD, and Terrence J. Sejnowski PhD. *Liars, Lovers, and Heroes.* NY:HarperCollins Publishers Inc., 2002. Padus, Emrika, Editor. *The Complete Guide to Your Emotions and Your Health.* PA:Rodale Press, 1986.

Protein (Accessed Jun, '16)
   https://ghr.nlm.nih.gov/primer/howgeneswork/protein

   http://www.health.harvard.edu/blog/how-much-protein-do-you-need-every-day-201506188096

Rabin, Roni Caryn. "For a Sharp Brain, Stimulation."
http://www.nytimes.com/2008/05/13/health/13brain.html?_r=2&em&ex=1211601600&en=d7a1026cb34907fd&ei=5087

Randall, David K. *Dreamland: Adventures in the Strange Science of Sleep.* NY:W.W. Norton and Company, Inc., 2012

Ratey, John J. MD. *A User's Guide to the Brain.* NY:Vintage Books, 2002.

Ratey, John J. MD, and Eric Hagerman. *Spark: The Revolutionary New Science of Exercise and the Brain.* NY:Little, Brown and Company, 2008.

Reiter, Russel, J., PhD, and Jo Robinson. *Melatonin: Your Body's Natural Wonder Drug.* NY:Bantam Books, 1995.

Restak, Richard, MD. *Mozart's Brain and the Fighter Pilot.* NY:Harmony Books, 2001.

_____. *Mysteries of the Mind.* Washingto.n, DC: National Geographic, 2000.

Roisen, Michael F., MD and Mehmet C. Oz, MD. *YOU: The Owner's Manual.* NY:William Morrow Paperbacks, 2013.

Roizen, Michael F., MD. *Real Age: Are You As Young As You Can Be?* NY:HarperCollins Publishers, 2001.
Rosen, Stephen. *Weathering: How the atmosphere conditions your body, your mind, your moods—and your health.* NY:M.Evans and Company Inc, 1979.

Rosenthal, Norman, E., MD. *The Emotional Revolution.* NY:Citadel Press, 2003.

_____. *Winter Blues. Revised Edition: Everything You Need to Know to Beat Seasonal Affective Disorder.* NY:Guilford Press, 2006.

Sapolsky, Robert M., PhD. *Why Zebras Don't Get Ulcers.* NY:W. H. Freeman and Company, 1994.

Schacter, Daniel L., PhD. *Searching For Memory: The Brain, The Mind, And The Past.* NY:Basic Books, 1997.

Schacter, Daniel L., PhD. *The Seven Sins of Memory: How the Mind Forgets and Remembers.* NY:Mariner Books, 2002.

Schwartz, Jeffrey M., MD, and Sharon Begley. *The Mind & the Brain.* NY:Regan Books, 2002.

Seaward, Brian Luke. *Achieving the Mind-Body-Spirit Connection: A Stress Management Workbook.* Boston:Jones and Bartlett Publishers Inc, 2004.

Segerberg, Osborn. Jr. *Living To Be 100.* NY:Charles Scribner's Sons, 1982.

Siebert, Al, PhD, with foreword by Bernie Siegel, MD. *The Survivor Personality.* NY:Perigee Books, 1996.

Siegel, Daniel J. *The Developing Mind.* NY:The Guilford Press, 1999.

Sies, Helmut, Editor. *Antioxidants in Disease Mechanisms and Illness.* UK:Academic Press, 1997.

Singh, Dalip, PhD. *Emotional Intelligence at Work.* NY:Sage, 2000.

Sloat, Donald E., PhD. *Growing Up Holy & Wholly.* TN:Wolgemuth & Hyatt Pub, 1990.

Small, Gary, MD. *The Memory Bible*. NY:Hyperion, 2002.

Snowdon, David, PhD. *Aging with Grace.* NY:Bantam Books, 2001.

Stine, Jean Marie. *Double Your Brain Power*. NY:Prentice Hall, Inc, 1997.

Stroebel, Charles F., MD. *QR - The Quieting Reflex.* NY:The Berkley Publishing Group, 1983.

Sylvia, Claire, with William Novak. *A Change of Heart.* NY:Little, Brown and Company, 1997.

Taylor, Arlene R. PhD, and W. Eugene Brewer, EdD. *Your Brain Has a Bent (Not a Dent!)* 3rd Edition.. CA:Success Resources International, 2009 and 2014.

Taylor, Arlene, R., PhD, Sharlet M. Briggs, PhD, and Steve Horton, MPH. *Longevity Lifestyle Matters—Keeping Your Brain, Body, and Weight in the Game.* CA:Success Resources International, 2015.

Taylor, Arlene, R., PhD, and Sharlet M. Briggs, PhD. *The Longevity Mystery Club.* CA:Success Resources International, 2015.

Taylor, Arlene, R., PhD, and Sharlet M. Briggs, PhD. *The Adventures of Aimi.* CA:Success Resources International, 2014.

Taylor, Arlene, R., PhD, and Sharlet M. Briggs, PhD. *The Adventures of Stella.* CA:Success Resources International, 2015.

Taylor, Arlene, R., PhD, and Sharlet M. Briggs, PhD. *Age-Proofing Your Memory—the Ultimate Brain Builder.* CA:Success Resources International, 2008.

Thomas, Pat. *Under the Weather: How Weather and Climate Affect Our Health.* VA:Vision, 2004.

Townsend, John, PhD. *Who's Pushing Your Buttons.* TN:Integrity Publishers, 2004.

Van Welleghen .L., et al. "Pre-meal Water Consumption Reduced Meal Energy Intake in Older but not Younger Subjects." Obesity. 15:93-97. 2007.)

Wegner, Daniel M., PhD. *White Bears and Other Unwanted Thoughts.* NY:The Guilford Press, 1994.

Waitley, Denis. *Seeds of Greatness.* NY:Pocket, 2988.

Wolpert, Stuart. 'Dieting Does Not Work, UCLA Researchers Report.' UCLA Newsroom. UCLA. (Accessed Dec, 2013)

Woods, Bob, et al. "Cognitive Stimulation to Improve Cognitive Functioning in People with Dementia." (http://www.ucl.ac.uk/international-cognitive-stimulation-therapy/publications/pdfs/woods-aguirre-spector-orrell-2011)

Yang, Sarah. "Lifelong brain-stimulating habits linked to lower Alzheimer's protein levels." (http://news.berkeley.edu/2012/01/23/engaged-brain-amyloid-alzheimers/)

Zander, Rosamund Stone, and Benjamin Zander. *The Art of Possibility: Transforming Professional and Personal Life.* NY:Penguin (Non-Classics), 2002.

Zull, James, E., PhD. *The Art of Changing the Brain.* Virginia:Stylus Publishing, LLC, 2002.

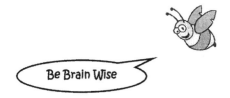

Be Brain Wise

The human body is programmed to last one or two decades past the century mark.

If you don't sabotage its natural process, your chances of making it to 120 are excellent.

—Walter M. Bortz II MD

Stanford University Clinical Associate Professor, and co-chair of the AMA-ANA Task Force on Aging

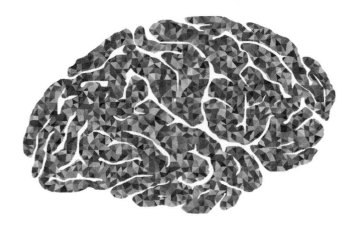

—The End—